T0259020

AN INTRODUCTION TO INCLUSIVE HEALTHCARE DESIGN

An Introduction to Inclusive Healthcare Design is a comprehensive guide to the design and facilitation of safe, healthy, equitable, and inclusive healthcare settings across a variety of scales. The book informs healthcare professionals, healthcare administrators, planners, designers in the healthcare sector, design students, and faculty about best practices and considerations for inclusive design.

The primary theme for the book is *design for all* – considering the design of healthcare spaces through the lenses of inclusivity and social equity. Part 1 presents the reader with an overview of the variety of locations and types of healthcare settings. Part 2 provides a comprehensive overview of the principles of equitable and inclusive healthcare design and considers how these principles can be applied to the range of settings laid out in Part 1. The authors consider inclusivity-supportive infrastructure in primary and ancillary spaces within healthcare settings. Part 3 envisions the future of inclusive healthcare design, considering the integration of virtual reality and artificial intelligence, as well as addressing the ever more relevant issue of healthcare provision in settings at risk of natural disasters.

Denise M. Linton is a retired tenured professor and professorship holder from the University of Louisiana at Lafayette. She is a former researcher, an international speaker, an author, and an active Fellow of the American Association of Nurse Practitioners.

Kiwana T. McClung is a professor in the School of Architecture & Design and serves as Chief Inclusion Officer at the University of Louisiana at Lafayette.

AN INTRODUCTION TO INCLUSIVE HEALTHCARE DESIGN

Edited by Denise M. Linton
and Kiwana T. McClung

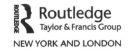

Routledge
Taylor & Francis Group

NEW YORK AND LONDON

Designed cover image: © Getty Images

First published 2025
by Routledge
605 Third Avenue, New York, NY 10158

and by Routledge
4 Park Square, Milton Park, Abingdon, Oxon, OX14 4RN

Routledge is an imprint of the Taylor & Francis Group, an informa business

Library of Congress Cataloging-in-Publication Data
Names: McClung, Kiwana T., editor. | Linton, Denise M., editor.
Title: An introduction to inclusive healthcare design / edited by Denise M. Linton,
    DNS, FNP, FAANP and Kiwana T. McClung, Assoc. AIA, NOMA.
Description: New York, NY : Routledge, 2024. | Includes bibliographical references
    and index.
Identifiers: LCCN 2023056865 (print) | LCCN 2023056866 (ebook) | ISBN
    9781032540481 (hbk) | ISBN 9781032540498 (pbk) | ISBN 9781003414902 (ebk)
Subjects: LCSH: Health facilities—Planning. | Health facilities—Design and
    construction. | Social medicine.
Classification: LCC RA967 .I624 2024 (print) | LCC RA967 (ebook) |
    DDC 362.1—dc23/eng/20240405
LC record available at https://lccn.loc.gov/2023056865
LC ebook record available at https://lccn.loc.gov/2023056866

ISBN: 978-1-032-54048-1 (hbk)
ISBN: 978-1-032-54049-8 (pbk)
ISBN: 978-1-003-41490-2 (ebk)

DOI: 10.4324/9781003414902

Typeset in Joanna
by Apex CoVantage, LLC

CONTENTS

CONTRIBUTORS

Kristi L. Anderson, PhD

Dr. Kristi L. Anderson, an experienced healthcare leader, researcher, and educator, is the University of Louisiana at Lafayette's chief strategy officer. In this role, she works with senior leadership to create and build visionary pathways, partnerships, and growth opportunities for the university.

Prior to joining the family, Dr. Anderson held several positions at LSU Health Sciences Center/University Hospital and Clinics in Lafayette, where she was an assistant professor of research in the Department of Medicine. She served as the campus ombudsman, director of graduate medical education, research coordinator, and created and chaired a grant program within LSU's School of Medicine for healthcare disparities and inequities. She enjoys studying barriers or gaps within systems and how to outfit systems with resources and connections that allow for transformational growth and development.

Dr. Anderson also has extensive experience in implementing initiatives related to diversity, equity, inclusion, and belonging (DEIB). She has consulted local hospitals on their DEIB programming and served as diversity and inclusion officer for the LSU Health Sciences Center/University Hospital and Clinics medical education programs. She's also presented public and academic lectures on the topic.

She serves on the Louisiana Health Works Commission and was appointed by Gov. John Bel Edwards to the state's COVID-19 Health Equity Task Force, to which she was honored with a Senate Resolution, No. 66. She was named the 2021–2022 Scholar in Residence for Dillard University's Minority Health and Health Disparities Center.

Dr. Anderson holds a PhD in systemic studies from the University of Louisiana at Monroe. She has taught at the California Institute of Integral Studies, Tulane University Medical School, San Francisco State University, and Southeastern Louisiana University.

Angela A. Appiah, PhD, DNP, MPH, RN, COA, FAACM

Dr. Appiah is a Fulbright Specialist and executive administrator for healthcare systems, and she has 25 years of healthcare experience. Her expertise is in health systems and services management consulting, program development, accreditation, undergraduate and graduate education, executive administrator for the oncology service line (acute and ambulatory), heart failure services, disease prevention/detection, health promotion, navigation, palliative care, and supportive programs such as navigation. As a clinical operations and research leader, she focuses on program development, sustainment, implementing science/translational research, and global population health.

Dr. Appiah is the founder and president of the Hudson Valley New York Black Nurses Association, Inc. (chartered chapter of NBNA.org). She is presently employed as an associate chief nursing officer at JJP VAMC. She has also been at Pace University since 2018, holding the title of adjunct associate professor at the College of Health Professions – Health Science Program & Lienhard School of Nursing. Dr. Appiah is also a consultant at St. Jude Children's Research Hospital (St. Jude Global) and founder and CEO of Global Population Health Consulting, LLC. She has worked with diverse countries' ministries of health and programs globally to build capacity and develop and sustain health systems.

Dr. Appiah's past experiences include executive administrator, AVP, and director positions. She is a fellow of numerous organizations: Fellow of the American Academy of Case Management (FAACM); American Organization for Nursing Leadership (AONL), previously known as the American Organization for Nurse Executives (AONE) and AONL Foundation Nurse Director Fellow; and AONE Aspiring Nurse Leaders fellow, Oncology Nursing Society (ONS) Leadership Development Institute.

She has developed and participated in numerous mentoring and coaching programs for diverse organizations. She participates in multiple professional organizations and recently co-authored a chapter on mentoring and coaching in the book *21st Century Nursing Leadership*, edited by Dr. Mary Gullatte. In addition, she has presented numerous times at conferences locally, nationally, and globally.

Dr. Appiah seeks to reduce the burden of preventable disease among populations of African descent in the United States and Africa through evidence-based quality improvement, community-engaged research, and implementation science.

She serves on numerous boards globally. Examples include the Oncology Nursing Society (ONS) Leadership Development Committee, Nurses on Boards Coalition State Contacts Co-Chair. She also serves on diverse committees as the co-chair/chair. She has received multiple awards and recognitions and recently won awards such as an honoree of the NYONL nurse executive rising star award for 2022 and AONL 2019 Young Professional Voices award for recognition and exhibition of exemplary leadership within her organization, community, and the nursing profession. Dr. Appiah was the 2019 National Black Nurses Association Administrative Nurse of the Year and the 40 under 40 awards. She also received the 2019 Oncology Nursing Society Foundation and the National Black Nurses Association doctoral scholarships.

Dr. Appiah feels her purpose is to transform global health systems, especially those in low-resource areas globally, contributing to healthcare through improving disease prevention, health promotion, mentoring, coaching, and sponsoring potential leaders.

Keneshia Bryant-Moore, PhD, APRN, FNP-BC

Dr. Bryant-Moore is a tenured professor in the Department of Health Behavior and Health Education at the University of Arkansas for Medical Sciences (UAMS) in the Fay W. Boozman College of Public Health. Presently, she serves as the Director of the Community Engagement and Dissemination Core of the Arkansas Center for Health Disparities (ARCHD) and Associate Director of the Community Engagement Core of the UAMS Translational Research Institute (TRI). In these roles, she provides resources to researchers on engaging communities throughout the research process, including the dissemination of research findings.

Dr. Bryant-Moore's research primarily focuses on health disparities and inequities experienced by minority racial/ethnic groups and rural and vulnerable populations. Over the past decade, her research has been in collaboration primarily with the faith community in Arkansas, which has led to the development of faith-based health interventions, programs, and other research endeavors. Also, to support the efforts of long-term engagement in research with the faith community, she has been awarded several contracts from the Patient-Centered Outcomes Research Institute (PCORI) to support research dissemination, training, and platforms to generate new research ideas. Through this support, she led the development of the Faith-Academic Initiative for Transforming Health (FAITH) Network in 2016. As part of this network faith leaders are educated on the basic principles of research and health-related issues and given the opportunity to partner in research and program efforts.

Dr. Bryant-Moore received her bachelor of science in nursing and bachelor of science in healthcare administration from the University of Michigan-Flint, her master of science in nursing from Duke University, and her PhD in nursing from Azusa Pacific University. Dr. Bryant-Moore is the mother of four daughters and enjoys traveling, dancing, singing, baking, and spending time with family and friends.

Beverly Ann Collins, RN, MS, CIC, FAPIC
Beverly Ann (Beverly) Collins has more than 30 years of experience in infection prevention and control (IPC) in acute and long-term care settings and is board certified in infection control (CIC) since 1992. She has achieved the highest infection prevention certification level as a fellow of the Association of Professionals in Infection Control and Epidemiology in 2017.

During her tenure in IPC, Collins has served at the director level for more than 20 years. She also has public health experience as a public health epidemiologist at the New York City Department of Health and Mental Hygiene (NYC DOHMH) Bureau of Communicable Disease. She has served as a core strategic member of the emergency preparedness program at a major teaching hospital, where she was instrumental in developing the biological response to emergencies. She also has experience on emergency preparedness committees at various hospitals as an active subject matter expert on tabletop and functional emergency preparedness drills.

From 2000 to 2012, Collins served on the Metropolitan Medical Response System (MMRS) committee for the city of Newark in New Jersey and on the regional Urban Area Security Initiative (UASI) committee in northern New Jersey during the same period. Her training in emergency preparedness includes Federal Emergency Management Administration (FEMA) incident command system courses levels 100, 200, 700, and 800 and certification as a FEMA-certified emergency preparedness trainer through course work at the Center for Domestic Preparedness in Anniston, Alabama. Her education includes a BA in biology, MS in microbiology and ASN in nursing.

Justin Fontenot, DNP, RN, NEA-BC, FAADN

Dr. Justin Fontenot is an assistant professor of nursing in the LHC Group Myers School of Nursing at the University of Louisiana at Lafayette. He is a board-certified nurse executive advanced. Before his academic career, Dr. Fontenot was a home care service delivery leader with a decade of experience from the roadside to the board room in varying roles and experiences. He is a fellow in the Academy of Associate Degree Nursing and the Editor-in-Chief of the academic peer-reviewed journal *Teaching and Learning in Nursing*. Dr. Fontenot teaches undergraduate community health clinical courses and has research expertise in teaching methods, VR simulation, LGBTQIA+ health equity, and clinical reasoning in nursing practice and education. He holds a master's in nursing administration and leadership, a doctorate in nursing practice, and is a current DNP to PhD in nursing science student at Texas Woman's University. He resides in South Louisiana.

Marianne Graffam, AIA, ACHA, NCIDQ, LEED AP BD+C, CHID, EDAC

Marianne Graffam is a senior associate and the director of health and wellness at EskewDumezRipple (EDR). She joined EDR with a focus on healthcare to augment and grow the firm's vision and body of work in the realm of health and wellness. Originally born in Seoul, South Korea, Marianne grew up in Ocala, Florida. After attending Tulane University School of Architecture and spending parts of her career in Seattle and Tacoma, Washington, and Honolulu, Hawaii, Marianne found a passion for working closely with healthcare stakeholders to create spaces that can aid users in providing the best possible care. She has achieved her certification as a healthcare architect through the American College of Healthcare Architects (ACHA), healthcare interior designer (CHID), and her evidence-based design accreditation and certification (EDAC).

She is a proud proponent of the belief that architecture and design should apply the scientific process to address design problems and question hypotheses to achieve outcomes that are aesthetically pleasing and functionally beautiful.

In the community, Marianne is active with the nonprofit unCommon Construction and engaged with the AIA at the local and state levels. Since 2009 she has also served as a city organizer for PechaKucha Nights in Tacoma and New Orleans with over 30 successful events.

Garold Hamilton, MSc (Dist.), BSc (Hons), PMP, CEng, PE, LEED AP, FASHE, CxA, EDAC

Garold Hamilton is the US Director of Healthcare and Senior Vice President for WSP, one of the world's largest engineering and infrastructure firms. He graduated from the University of the West Indies with an Upper Second Class Honors Degree and graduated from South Bank University in London with a master's degree in mechanical engineering, with distinction. He is a licensed professional engineer in the United States as well as in Europe. He has over 25 years of experience in the design and construction of healthcare facilities all over the world. He was elevated to fellow status for the American Hospital Association. He is a healthcare thought leader and has over 40 articles in multiple healthcare and engineering publications. He is also a seasoned presenter and has presented nationally and internationally at several conferences and seminars. His work has been recognized with several design honors, including most recently the ASHRAE Technology 1st Place Award for Healthcare Engineering Design. In 2015 he was named 40 under 40 by the *Consulting-Specifying Engineer Magazine* for engineers who stand out in a variety of personal and professional aspects in their lives.

In 2006, he founded the IRS-approved 501(c)(3) nonprofit organization Dreams to Reality Foundation (DTR Foundation), a broad-based community initiative that assists low-income children to complete their education and achieve economic self-sufficiency through sports. He is also an author of the inspirational novel *Ghetto Youths' Bible*. In addition, he is a motivational speaker and speaks at school graduations, conferences, and webinars.

Alexander Lazard, BSUSP, ABA

Alexander Lazard seamlessly merges business acumen with community dedication. Boasting over a decade of experience, he has honed his skills in operations optimization and crafting strategic plans for renowned community organizations. Lazard's expertise lies in making visionary decisions that bolster business and community, forging strategies for equity optimization, and meticulously crafting efficient yet robust processes.

As a Lafayette native, he has garnered recognition, notably the Top 20 Under 40 Acadiana Young Leader Award. He holds significant roles across Louisiana, such as administrative pastor at Destiny of Faith Church, urban planner for Lafayette Consolidated Government, board chair at Leadership Institute of Acadiana, board chair at Evangeline Thruway Redevelopment Team, and numerous leadership positions in local organizations. His academic credentials include a ministry certificate, an associate in business administration (Northwestern State University), and a bachelor's in urban studies and planning (University of New Orleans), with research in environmental justice (Michigan State University) and coastal ecosystem design (Louisiana State University).

Lazard functions with a unique blend of visionary zeal and economic pragmatism, managing partnerships and driving community projects, working closely with neighborhood groups, promoting healthy urban designs, and fostering local community spirit. Lazard consistently navigates multifaceted challenges, emphasizing advocacy, strategic foresight, and adaptability.

Christy Lenahan, DNP, FNP-BC, ENP-C, CNE

Dr. Lenahan is an associate professor in the LHC Group Myers School of Nursing at the University of Louisiana at Lafayette and serves as the graduate nursing coordinator. She is board certified as a family and emergency nurse practitioner and certified nurse educator. Dr. Lenahan has mentored and assisted several students and community partners with research focused on improving patient outcomes, including the use of remote patient monitoring. She actively practices with a current focus on HIV prevention and treatment as well as aesthetic medicine.

Denise M. Linton, DNS, FNP, FAANP

Dr. Linton is a retired tenured professor and professorship holder from the University of Louisiana at Lafayette. She is a former researcher, an international speaker, an author, and an active fellow of the American Association of Nurse Practitioners. Dr. Linton's healthcare profession and service span more than three decades. She earned her doctor of nursing science (DNS) degree from Louisiana State University Health Sciences Center – New Orleans in 2009; master of science in nursing and family nurse practitioner certificate from Columbia University in New York in 1999; bachelor of science in nursing from Medgar Evers College, Brooklyn, New York, in 1996, and diploma in nursing from University Hospital of the West Indies School of Nursing in 1986.

Jessica McCarthy, DNP, MHSA, MSN, APRN, FNP-BC

Dr. McCarthy is a University of Louisiana at Lafayette graduate, where she earned her bachelor of science in nursing and her master of science in nursing. She also earned her master's in health service administration from the University of St. Francis in Illinois and her doctorate in nursing practice from the University of Alabama-Huntsville. She has been an RN for over 30 years, a family nurse practitioner for over 15 years, and a nurse educator for over 12 years. Currently she is an associate professor at Chamberlain University working within the DNP program. She has conducted research in the field of domestic violence and has published numerous articles on the subject. She has also presented on local, state, and national levels on the topic of domestic violence. She continues to research and publish on domestic violence while also educating the public and professionals on this pertinent issue facing us today. In addition, she continues to research and publish on public health areas, including current infections affecting communities locally, nationally, and worldwide.

Kiwana T. McClung, Assoc. AIA, NOMA

Kiwana T. McClung is a professor in the School of Architecture & Design and serves as Chief Inclusion Officer at the University of Louisiana at Lafayette. In this role, she is responsible for fostering diversity among students, faculty, and staff, as well as ensuring that underrepresented groups have equal access to educational opportunities and resources. Prior to joining the faculty at UL Lafayette, Kiwana worked as an architectural designer for several firms around South Louisiana. A graduate of Louisiana State University's School of Architecture and Design, Kiwana is regionally and nationally recognized for her leadership, research, and efforts toward increasing diversity within a school of architecture and curricula.

Elham Morshedzadeh, Ph.D.

Elham Morshedzadeh, Ph.D., is an industrial designer, usability researcher, and educator whose research focuses on healthcare, community-centered design, and usability. She has taught design internationally and in the US, and was recently honored with the 2021 Young Educator Award from the Industrial Designers Society of America (IDSA).

Since 2017, she has collaborated with clinicians, engineers, and faculty to create unique research and design initiatives in telehealth, healthcare, and public health, many of which have been funded by various organizations such as the National Institutes of Health (NIH), and the Office of National Drug Control Policy (ONDCP). Dr. Morshedzadeh has cultivated distinctive learning experiences for her students through their engagement in healthcare design.

Before entering academia, Dr. Morshedzadeh spent a decade as a professional industrial designer in Iran, where she served as the lead designer on a range of high-profile Design projects. Her classroom teaching integrates her extensive industry experience, and her collaborations with engineers, anthropologists, and scientists. Her pedagogical approach underscores the importance of experiential, evidence-based decision-making in participatory design with an emphasis on community engagement.

Dr. Morshedzadeh serves as the South District representative for the Women in Design Committee within the IDSA, collaborating with fellow committee members to enhance opportunities for female and non-binary designers. In August 2022, she joined the University of Houston as a Presidential Frontiers Assistant Professor for Healthcare Innovation.

Harmony Rochon, MS, EdD

Dr. Harmony Rochon is a native of Cecilia, Louisiana. She completed her bachelor's degree in psychology at Louisiana State University, her master's in psychology at Pennsylvania State University, and finished her doctor of education degree at University of Louisiana, Lafayette in 2017. Dr. Rochon is a licensed emergency medical technician and works as the Assistant Dean of Allied Health at South Louisiana Community College. She leads the following departments: Medical Assistants, Medical Lab Sciences, and Paramedics.

Dr. Rochon is a former LSU Golden Girl and New Orleans Saintsation. She is married to cardiologist and philanthropist Dr. Brent Rochon, and they live in Lafayette, Louisiana, with their sons Lloyd and Lawrence and their dog Luna.

Kari J. Smith, M Arch

Kari J. Smith is an academic professional, currently a professor of architecture and holding the position of interim associate dean of the College of the Arts at the University of Louisiana at Lafayette. Driven by a passion for architecture and a commitment to transdisciplinary problem-solving, Smith has an established record focused on coastal resilience and sustainable design.

Smith's education culminated in attaining the master of architecture, the terminal degree, from Rice University in 2005. Her academic pursuits have laid the foundation for a career marked by research excellence and a commitment to addressing critical challenges through collaborative efforts.

Her contributions to projects funded by the Department of Energy, Federal Highway Administration/Louisiana Department of Transportation and Development, Louisiana Board of Regents Enhancement Grant, and National Science Foundation Water Sustainability and Climate, as well as her record of publications and exhibitions, reflect a commitment to address complex issues, characterized by innovative solutions and a dedication to fostering resilience in the face of environmental challenges. Smith and other team members hold a U.S. Design Patent (patent number US D910,873 S, granted on February 16, 2021).

Twila Sterling-Guillory, PhD, APRN, FNP-BC

Dr. Sterling-Guillory received a bachelor of science degree in nursing from McNeese State University in 1993 and a master of science in nursing with a family nurse practitioner focus in 1998 from McNeese State University. She earned a PhD in nursing research from Southern A&M University in Baton Rouge, Louisiana, in 2011.

She has practiced as a nurse practitioner in several different clinical settings. She is currently practicing as a nurse practitioner in the hospice setting. She was promoted to the rank of professor in the College of Nursing and Health Professions in spring of 2021. She was the first African American faculty member in the College of Nursing and Health Professions to be promoted to this rank in the 65-year history of the college. In the spring of 2021, she was the first African American professor to be promoted to the position of program coordinator of the Graduate Nursing Program, and in the fall of 2023, she was the first African American professor to be promoted to department head of the Graduate Nursing Program at McNeese State University.

Dr. Sterling-Guillory is a member of Sigma Theta Tau International and Alpha Kappa Alpha Sorority, Inc.

Ronnie Ursin, DNP, MBA, RN, CENP, FACHE

Dr. Ronnie Ursin is a native of New Orleans, Louisiana. He is a healthcare executive and professional registered nurse with 20 years of experience in the health services. His clinical experience includes medical-surgical, telemetry, oncology, and cardiac, medical, and surgical intensive care. He is certified as a nurse executive and a Fellow in the American College of Healthcare Executives.

Dr. Ursin holds an associate degree in nursing from the Los Angeles Trade-Technical College; bachelor of science in public health from Dillard University; bachelor of science in nursing, master of science – health services leadership and management, and post-master certificate in teaching in nursing and health professions from the University of Maryland, Baltimore; master of business administration from Hood College; and doctor of nursing practice from Case Western Reserve University.

Dr. Ursin has held several executive leadership roles in small to large acute care hospitals as chief executive officer and chief nursing officer. He currently serves as adjunct faculty at the University of Maryland-Baltimore.

Dr. Ursin has made a significant impact on the healthcare community in the following past and current roles: He is currently the President-elect and Treasurer for the Association of Black Nursing Faculty (ABNF), treasurer of the ABNF Foundation, board member for the Eastern Pennsylvania Healthcare Executive Network, board member and officer of the National Black Nurses Association (NBNA), president of the Black Nurses Association of Baltimore, manuscript reviewer for the *Journal of Adult Health*; advisory board member of *Minority Nurse Magazine*; and board member of the National Coalition of Ethnic Minority Nurse Associations.

Christian Wild, EMT

Christian Wild has been working in the field of emergency medical services since 2014 as an emergency medical technician with Acadian Ambulance. In 2015 he became a nationally registered and state-licensed paramedic, completing his associate of applied science degree at South Louisiana Community College.

Wild lives and works in the New Orleans metro area in advanced life support, where he is currently a full-time community paramedic employed by Acadian Health. He also enjoys teaching new EMTs and was employed as a full-time EMT instructor with the National EMS Academy from 2020 to 2023; he now volunteers at the New Orleans NEMSA location teaching EMT skills to new students.

Veronica D. Woodard, PhD

Dr. Veronica D. Woodard is a retired associate professor from the College of Nursing & Health Professions at McNeese State University. She amassed an impressive 40 years in the profession of nursing prior to retirement. After earning an undergraduate bachelor of science in nursing degree from Dillard University, she continued her education, receiving a master of nursing degree from Louisiana State University Medical Center-Graduate School of Nursing, which is now Louisiana State University Health Sciences Center. Dr Woodard pursued and obtained the doctor of philosophy degree in education from Duplichain University.

She was recently certified as a faith community nurse by Baptist Community Ministries in April 2022. Dr. Woodard has experience in different capacities, including entrepreneurship as a home health agency owner for 10 years, clinical nurse specialist, and educator.

Part 1

OVERVIEW OF THE VARIETY OF SCALES, LOCATIONS, AND TYPES OF HEALTHCARE SETTINGS

1

REGIONAL HEALTHCARE SYSTEMS

Garold Hamilton

Regional hospitals or district hospitals serve a wider geographical region than a local or rural one, and in some countries, they define specific services that they are required to provide. Regional healthcare systems refer to an association of healthcare facilities and providers who collaborate to provide medical care and services to residents in an assigned geographical region (Definitive Healthcare, 2023) (Ramos et al. 2020). These systems include hospitals, clinics, rehabilitation centers, long-term care facilities, and other healthcare providers that deliver coordinated, comprehensive, and high-quality care across various locations and specialties (Medstar Health, 2023a, 2023b, 2023c). They may also be responsible for managing population healthcare needs, implementing relevant policies and programs, and guaranteeing access to essential healthcare services for all of their constituents. By working together, healthcare providers can share resources, knowledge, and expertise to better serve the recipients of healthcare services (Medstar Health, 2023a). Integration provides patient-centric care by bringing together services and processes into one cohesive whole, helping patients

DOI: 10.4324/9781003414902-2

navigate providers within a region more easily and manage their own care needs (National Academies of Sciences, Engineering, and Medicine, 2021)

Healthcare systems throughout the world vary considerably in philosophy and structure, yet all share one goal – to deliver top-quality care in each of the areas they serve (Ramos et al., 2020). At its core, healthcare delivery should provide high-quality care at affordable costs to all consumers. Unfortunately, rising healthcare costs remain an intractable challenge that many countries struggle to contain. Healthcare systems strive to offer care of the highest quality at an accessible cost and ensure environmental sustainability. On an international scale, U.S. healthcare spending made up approximately 17.8% of gross domestic product (GDP) in 2021 (Gunja et al., 2023). This is an immense problem, as many underserved communities still lack access to proper healthcare services. This was made evident during the COVID-19 pandemic where these communities were more severely impacted and led to an increased death toll (Gunja et al., 2023). Black people, comprising 45% of the District of Columbia's population, made up an estimated 75% of coronavirus deaths in that district (Moore, 2022). Hispanic people were also overrepresented, but not by much; 28% of cases, 13 deaths, and 11% of the population fell into their category (Hill, 2022).

Nations such as the UK and Canada with universal healthcare systems had long prioritized access by shortening wait times, but more recently have switched focus and are prioritizing sustainability and smart healthcare services (NHS, 2019). Establishing a healthcare system capable of meeting these challenges is no simple feat; however, taking a regional approach to healthcare delivery has proven successful for many healthcare systems in the United States, producing significant advantages over many single facilities.

Types of Regional Healthcare Systems

There are various regional healthcare systems, each offering unique characteristics and specializations. Examples are:

1. Academic medical centers: Academic medical centers are regional healthcare systems that are associated with medical schools or universities that focus on research, education, and patient care (Shi & Singh, 2022). These centers typically offer specialized services that are provided

by highly experienced healthcare providers and that boast cutting-edge research that often results in groundbreaking innovations and treatments (Association of American Medical Colleges [AAMC], 2023).

2. Community health systems: Community health systems are regional healthcare systems that are dedicated to serving underserved populations. Usually located in rural areas, they comprise healthcare providers who specialize in primary care services, preventive healthcare measures, and disease management. Additionally, these systems work closely with community organizations and local governments to meet unique healthcare requirements within their respective communities (United States Agency for International Development, n.d.).

3. Hospital systems: Hospital systems are regional healthcare networks with multiple hospitals and healthcare facilities within an area. These hospitals and facilities offer emergency, specialty, primary, and preventative healthcare services to residents in that geographic region. Hospital systems will often boast extensive networks of providers offering advanced treatments and technologies (AAMC, 2023).

4. Managed care organizations: Managed care organizations (MCOs) are regional healthcare systems that are dedicated to managing the health needs of specific populations. MCOs contract with healthcare providers for services that they offer to their members and seek to control costs while improving care quality for members (Heaton & Tadi, 2023).

Advantages of a Good Regional Healthcare System

An efficient regional healthcare system offers several advantages for both patients and providers alike because it facilitates seamless care delivery and access. According to Barry et al. (2021), some key benefits associated with great regional healthcare systems are:

1. Expanded access to care: Regional healthcare systems offer patients greater access to medical care services in underserved communities where health resources may be limited.

2. Coordinated care: Regional healthcare systems offer integrated and comprehensive healthcare to their patients across locations and specialties. Consequently, fragmentation is decreased while simultaneously increasing the quality of care that is delivered.

3. Greater efficiency: By working collaboratively, healthcare providers can share resources, knowledge, and expertise to maximize efficiency while decreasing costs.

4. Improved patient outcomes: A successful healthcare system in any region can contribute to enhanced patient outcomes such as reduced hospital readmission rates and lower mortality rates.

5. Increased patient satisfaction: Those receiving care through regional healthcare systems often report higher levels of satisfaction. This is usually because of easier access to care, receiving clear communication updates more promptly, and having coordinated health care available.

6. Professional growth opportunities: Healthcare providers working within regional healthcare systems may find numerous opportunities for professional growth and collaboration with colleagues from different specializations and locations (Barry et al., 2021).

Overall, an outstanding regional healthcare system can have an immense positive effect on the communities it serves by offering coordinated, comprehensive, and high-quality care to patients.

Global Exemplars of Regional Healthcare Systems

Some global examples of regional healthcare systems are discussed next. It is apparent that they have similarities and differences and that they often seek to overcome barriers to providing high-quality health to all.

Regional Healthcare Systems in the United States

In the United States, healthcare is a complex multilayered system consisting of both public and private providers/insurers/insureds (Shi & Singh, 2022). Notably, this healthcare system does not fall under nationalization, and as a result only limited involvement from the federal government exists when managing the services that are provided. Most healthcare services in the United States are provided through hospitals, clinics, and practitioners – from hospitals and clinics that serve the poor to clinics that offer healthcare to those who can afford it. Private health insurance plans are available for purchase by individuals or families or their employees; they cover part of the costs involved with receiving healthcare services.

Public healthcare systems are managed largely through federal programs such as the Children's Health Insurance Program (CHIP), Medicare, and Medicaid. CHIP provides healthcare services to children, while Medicare offers healthcare coverage to people aged 65 years old or above as well as those with certain disabilities. Medicaid offers coverage to low-income individuals and families. In addition to these public programs, the U.S. government provides healthcare services to military members through the Department of Veterans Affairs (Shi & Singh, 2022).

The U.S. healthcare system is widely considered one of the costliest worldwide. And it faces numerous difficulties, such as limited access for low-income and uninsured individuals as well as rising healthcare costs and shortages in certain regions. There have been efforts underway to address these challenges, including expanding public healthcare programs and creating innovative payment models designed to reduce costs while improving care quality. Yet the U.S. healthcare system remains contentious, and debate about the best ways to ensure access to affordable yet high-quality healthcare is ongoing (Shi & Singh, 2022).

MedStar Regional Healthcare System

MedStar Regional Healthcare System is a nonprofit community-based healthcare system operating throughout Maryland, Virginia, and Washington, DC (Medstar Health, 2023a). The system serves millions annually as a nonprofit healthcare network that comprises ten hospitals as well as numerous outpatient facilities with thousands of staff. MedStar Regional Healthcare System offers comprehensive primary, specialty, and emergency healthcare services across an extensive spectrum of fields that range from primary care, specialty care, and emergency response, cancer care, cardiology, orthopedics, neurology, pediatrics, and women's health (Medstar Health, 2023b, 2023c). The system's commitment to high-quality healthcare, diversity, equity, and inclusion is evident by its many recognitions and awards (Medstar Health, 2023d).

This healthcare system is known for providing patient-centric care and improving community health in its service area. The system works closely with local organizations and leaders to address identified health needs within each neighborhood it serves. Furthermore, MedStar Regional Healthcare System takes pride in furthering medical research and education, working alongside academic institutions to train the next generation of healthcare providers while conducting groundbreaking studies that enhance patient outcomes (Medstar Health, 2023b).

Kaiser Permanente Regional Healthcare System

Kaiser Permanente is a nonprofit integrated healthcare system (Kaiser Permanente, 2023a) that operates throughout California, Colorado, Georgia, Hawaii, Maryland, Virginia, Oregon, Washington, and Washington, DC (Kaiser Permanente, 2023c). Kaiser Permanente offers comprehensive healthcare services including primary, specialty, and hospital care as well as preventive services for its members. Their services are provided through health maintenance organization (HMO) plans and Medicare Advantage plans in addition to healthcare plans that include HMO and preferred provider organization (PPO) combination plans.

Kaiser Permanente Healthcare System is known for its integrated model of care that prioritizes prevention and early identification of illnesses (Kaiser Permanente, 2023b). Kaiser's care delivery model features team-based care with physicians, nurses, pharmacists, and other healthcare professionals working collaboratively to deliver coordinated patient care. Kaiser uses advanced technologies such as electronic health records for seamless communication among providers as they coordinate care services for patients.

Kaiser Permanente is dedicated to improving the health of the communities that it serves and addressing the social determinants of health and wellness (Kaiser Permanente, 2023a). Working closely with local organizations and community leaders, Kaiser Permanente collaborates on efforts that identify health disparities, expanding access to care while investing in research to further advance medical knowledge and improve patient outcomes.

Kaiser Permanente stands out among healthcare providers with its integrated care delivery model, which places an emphasis on prevention and early detection services, and its dedication to improving community health (Kaiser Permanente, n.d.). As an organization, they focus on "a workplace for all"; consequently, the race, ethnicity, gender, and age of their employees reflect their diverse communities. They have received numerous diversity and inclusion awards that include the best place to work in the areas of LGBTQ+ equality and disability inclusion for 16 and 6 consecutive years, respectively (Kaiser Permanente, n.d.).

Canadian Regional Healthcare System

The Canadian regional healthcare system is generally publicly funded and run by provinces and territories, with some variations depending on each jurisdiction (Government of Canada, 2021; Tikkanen et al., 2020). Some key examples include funding, services that are covered, wait times, access to primary care services, private healthcare options, and governance. Each province and territory employs their own funding model for healthcare services.

Although every province and territory offers coverage for medically necessary services, what's covered can differ. Additionally, access to primary care services and wait times can differ significantly across provinces and territories for different procedures or services. For example, some provinces lack primary care specialists, while others have implemented strategies to expand access (Government of Canada, 2021; Ross University School of Medicine, 2023; Tickkanen et al., 2020). Some Canadians purchase private health insurance for services, such as dental care, that are not provided by the Canadian healthcare system (Ross University School of Medicine, 2023; Tikkanen et al., 2020).

There are variations across provinces and territories, but there are a few consistent features. These features are universal healthcare coverage, provincial/territorial health insurance plans, access to primary care, private healthcare options in Canada, and wait times for services. Canadian citizens and permanent residents can take advantage of universally funded health coverage to access essential services, including doctor visits, hospital stays, and diagnostic testing, at no extra charge. Each province and territory offers publicly funded health insurance plans, which provide medically necessary services at reasonable costs to its population. The services are typically funded by taxes and other government revenues. Canadians have access to primary healthcare services, which enable them to effectively manage and prevent illness. While Canada's healthcare system is generally consistent, coverage between provinces and territories can differ. For example, some may provide for certain prescription drugs while others do not.

Although healthcare services in Canada are mainly publicly funded, there are also private options such as private health insurance plans, clinics, and for-profit hospitals available that offer private healthcare solutions. Wait times for healthcare services can sometimes present an obstacle, especially for healthcare by a specialist (Tickkanen et al., 2020).

Overall, Canada's healthcare system strives to offer universal publicly funded coverage, with primary and preventative services as a priority. While variations exist between provinces and territories, which may cause some variance in province-to-province coverage levels, overall, its goal remains the same. Canadians generally benefit from accessing high-quality health services.

Regional Healthcare Systems in the UK

In the United Kingdom, healthcare services are managed under a publicly funded system known as the National Health Service (NHS) (NHS, 2021). Healthcare is administered by the Department of Health and Social Care and comprises both primary and secondary health services free of cost to all legal residents living within its boundaries.

The UK primary healthcare services are delivered by a network of general practitioners (GPs) and community health centers that specialize in preventative healthcare, health promotion, and treating common illnesses. GPs act as the first point of contact with their patients before referring them on to additional healthcare specialists as needed. Secondary healthcare in the UK is provided through hospitals, which specialize in treating more complicated medical conditions with specialist medical care and treatments. The NHS operates an extensive network of hospitals throughout Britain; larger ones can usually be found near major urban hubs. Additionally, the NHS provides dental and optometry care, mental healthcare services, and general practice consultation.

The NHS is funded through general taxation and national insurance contributions and operates on the principle of providing healthcare that is free at the point of use. Private healthcare facilities exist, though typically they're only utilized by those able to afford more costly medical treatments.

Overall, the NHS is widely respected for providing accessible, high-quality healthcare services that are inclusive to all UK residents regardless of ability to pay. Unfortunately, its system faces numerous challenges, such as an increasing demand for services, rising costs, and workforce shortages However, efforts are currently being undertaken in response to these obstacles to ensure that it continues to offer high-quality services to the UK population (NHS, 2021).

Jamaica's Healthcare System

Jamaica's healthcare system is funded and overseen primarily by its Ministry of Health and Wellness, with a combination of both public and private facilities contributing services (Expat Financial, n.d.; MOHW, n.d.). Its public healthcare system serves as the main provider for health services and includes hospitals, health centers, and clinics that deliver primary, secondary, and tertiary healthcare services throughout Jamaica. Larger hospitals are clustered near major urban centers. Primary healthcare services are delivered via a network of community health centers and clinics that specialize in preventive healthcare, health promotion, and treating common illnesses. Secondary and tertiary healthcare are typically delivered in hospitals which specialize in more focused care for complex medical conditions.

Jamaica's private healthcare system is relatively limited and focused mainly on those who can afford private medical treatment. This system includes private hospitals, clinics, and practitioners who offer their services at reasonable costs to individuals who are able to pay (Expat Financial, n.d.; MOHW, n.d.).

Overall, Jamaica's healthcare system faces numerous obstacles, including worker shortages, infrastructural issues, and equipment issues, as well as high rates of noncommunicable diseases such as diabetes, hypertension, and cancer. Efforts are being undertaken to overcome these hurdles, to enhance both accessibility and quality services provided to all Jamaicans.

South Africa's Healthcare System

South Africa's healthcare system consists of an intricate network of both public and private facilities providing healthcare to their populations (Conmy, 2018). They employ a two-tier healthcare model: public healthcare for most population segments, while those able to pay can opt for private medical attention.

Public healthcare services are administered by the government through its Department of Health (DOH) (Conmy, 2018). Hospitals, clinics, and community health centers operate under the purview of the DOH to provide primary, secondary, and tertiary healthcare to their populations. Tax revenues help fund this system that offers free or low-cost care options to those who can't afford private medical coverage. Private healthcare systems operate under market pressures and typically consist of hospitals, clinics, and practitioners catering exclusively to those able to pay (Conmy, 2018).

The South African healthcare system faces various difficulties. These difficulties range from shortages in workers and infrastructure/equipment needs to communicable/noncommunicable disease burden. Efforts are being undertaken to combat these difficulties and increase both access and quality in services for all South Africans.

The Benefits of Regional Healthcare Systems

It is apparent that regional healthcare systems play a vital role in healthcare delivery systems. They provide healthcare services directly to their communities and strive to enhance health and well-being among populations within these regions. Some roles of regional healthcare systems include:

1. Delivery of healthcare services: Regional healthcare systems provide their communities with a wide variety of healthcare services, such as primary, specialty, emergency, and preventive healthcare services. These systems strive to offer high-quality services at prices they can afford while being accessible and affordable for residents in their respective regions.
2. Support of local economies: Regional healthcare systems are often one of the largest employers in their respective regions because they create jobs, recruit skilled healthcare providers, and contribute to local economies. Furthermore, regional healthcare systems help attract businesses by offering quality healthcare services in their communities.
3. Health disparities reduction: Regional healthcare systems strive to reduce health disparities within their communities by offering healthcare services to underserved populations and addressing social determinants of health. They aim to promote optimal community health by making services affordable and accessible.
4. Medical research enhancement: Regional healthcare systems often partner with medical schools or universities and are known for their innovative research efforts, clinical trials, research regarding new treatments, and expanding medical knowledge. Regional healthcare systems play an essential role in furthering medical research while simultaneously improving quality-of-care standards for their respective patient populations.

Creating a Regional Healthcare System

Regional healthcare systems have a record of improving the quality of healthcare for their residents. However, creating a regional healthcare system is no simple task; here are a few steps that may be taken to begin the creation of such an entity:

1. *Conduct a needs analysis:* Begin by performing an in-depth needs analysis that assesses both community healthcare requirements and gaps within existing healthcare systems. This helps to pinpoint services or specialties that might be needed as well as where they should be located. This step can provide invaluable information.
2. *Engage stakeholders:* Involve and solicit feedback from all key healthcare stakeholders such as providers, community organizations, local government bodies, and private-sector partners as you establish the regional healthcare system. A steering committee or task force should then oversee the process of development.
3. *Plan the system:* Develop a strategic plan for a regional healthcare system that includes goals, objectives, and action steps designed to meet identified needs. Additionally, consider factors like staffing levels, technology investments, funding streams, and infrastructure. Planning and design professionals should be included in every step of this process to ensure that design considerations and parameters are clearly understood and addressed to the benefit of all.
4. *Form partnerships:* Work toward forging alliances between healthcare providers and organizations within the community. Seek funding opportunities from government, philanthropic, or private sources.
5. *Implement the plan:* Begin to put your plan into action by developing infrastructure, hiring staff, and forging partnerships with healthcare providers to establish access and affordability as primary goals of the system. Work hard to make sure everyone can afford and utilize this solution for healthcare purposes in your community.
6. *Monitor and evaluate:* Regularly monitor and evaluate the regional healthcare system to make sure it's meeting community needs and adjust as necessary to improve access, quality, and efficiency.
7. *Conduct post-occupancy evaluations:* Observing how healthcare system facilities operate and perform, individually and as components of the entire system, could provide a wealth of knowledge concerning inefficiencies and gaps in providing care. This will allow the appropriate adaptations and changes to be made in a timely manner.

Establishing a regional healthcare system may seem an impossible feat, yet with careful planning, stakeholder involvement, inclusive design strategies, and strategic partnerships, it can become a reality. A system that offers superior healthcare will bring greater community well-being.

The Role of Design Firms in the Establishment of Regional Healthcare Systems

Design firms play an invaluable role in creating successful regional healthcare systems by offering expertise in designing physical spaces, technology infrastructure, and patient experiences necessary for optimal healthcare (Brown & Smith, 2019). Design firms specialize in space planning for healthcare facilities such as hospitals and clinics. They do so to meet both patients' and providers' needs for functionality, efficiency, and aesthetics.

Healthcare systems may seek assistance from design firms to create technology infrastructure – for example, to equip electronic medical records (EMRs) and telemedicine platforms with user-friendly features that connect components securely. Design firms can also play an essential part in shaping patient experiences by designing waiting areas, signage, wayfinding, and other elements within the environment/space. They can incorporate lighting elements, furniture, fixtures, and equipment that are not only conducive to the physical health but also the mental well-being of patients. Their services can create spaces that are welcoming and promote healing for all of their clients. Additionally, healthcare facilities relying on design firms can enlist their assistance with creating energy-efficient and environmentally responsible facilities that minimize waste while simultaneously cutting energy consumption and increasing resiliency over time. They ensure designs adhere to best practices to reduce energy use while simultaneously encouraging sustainability. Finally, design firms also offer project management services to ensure healthcare systems are designed and constructed on schedule and within budget (Brown & Smith, 2019).

Design firms play an essential role when developing regional healthcare systems. They provide expertise to ensure physical spaces, technology infrastructure, and patient experiences all contribute to providing high-quality care services.

Conclusion

Regional healthcare systems play a vital role in providing patient-centric care and improving community health across different nations, such as the United States, Canada, the UK, Jamaica, and South Africa. By joining forces, regional systems bring healthcare facilities and providers from within a specific geographical area together in providing coordinated, comprehensive healthcare to residents within that geographic region. By working collaboratively on behalf of patients, these systems can share resources, expertise, and knowledge for improved access, efficiency, and patient outcomes.

U.S. healthcare systems are intricate, multilayered affairs composed of public and private providers, insurers, and insured individuals. While efforts have been undertaken to address challenges like rising healthcare costs and limited access for low-income individuals, debate surrounding this system continues. Canada's healthcare system aims for universal coverage, with each province and territory providing publicly funded health insurance plans that offer universal coverage; although coverage and wait times may differ between regions, overall, the goal remains the same – offering high-quality healthcare services to every citizen of this nation. The NHS in the UK offers free healthcare to legal residents. Funding comes largely through taxation; with this method the NHS aims to deliver accessible and inclusive care services across its scope of provision. Jamaica's healthcare system features both public and private facilities, with public services acting as its main provider. South Africa's healthcare system utilizes a two-tier model, offering free public healthcare to the majority of the population while private care options exist for those able to pay. Furthermore, traditional healers play an active part in rural healthcare provision, and this recognition extends even into private healthcare provision.

Regional healthcare systems across countries face many obstacles; nonetheless, efforts are ongoing to enhance access and quality of care for residents. By collaborating with design firms for their expertise, adopting cutting-edge technology solutions, and engaging stakeholders as a group in collaborations between them all, regional healthcare systems are constantly adapting and evolving in response to community needs. They play an essential role in supporting population health and well-being as they work toward meeting goals of providing high-quality yet cost-effective healthcare services to all.

References

Association of American Medical Colleges. (2023). *Building a systems approach to community health and health equity for academic health centers.* Retrieved October 4, 2023, from www.aamchealthjustice.org/resources/health-equity-systems

Barry, D., Yellen, E., & Chambers, N. (2021). Advantages of a good regional healthcare system. In *The handbook of healthcare management research* (pp. 253–266). Routledge.

Brown, P., & Smith, J. (2019). How can a design firm assist in establishing a regional healthcare system? In *Healthcare facility planning* (pp. 87–98). Springer.

Conmy, A. (2018). South African health care system analysis. *Public Health Review, 1(1).*

Definitive Healthcare. (2023). *Top 10 health systems in the U.S.* Retrieved August 24, 2023, from www.definitivehc.com

Expat Financial. (n.d.). *Jamaica healthcare system & medical insurance options for expats.* Retrieved August 16, 2023, from https://expatfinancial.com/healthcare-information-by-region/caribbean-healthcare-system/jamaica-healthcare-system/

Government of Canada. (2021). *Health care in Canada: Access our universal health care system.* Government of Canada. Retrieved August 5, 2023.

Gunja, M. Z., Gumas, E. D., & Williams, R. D., II (2023, January). *U.S. health care from a global perspective, 2022: Accelerating spending, worsening outcomes.* Commonwealth Fund. https://doi.org/10.26099/8ejy-yc74

Heaton, J., & Tadi, P. (2023, January). *Managed care organization – Statpearls – NCBI bookshelf.* National Library of Medicine, National Center for Biotechnology Information. https://ncbi.nlm.nih.gov/books/NBK557797/#!po=8.33333

Hill, L., & Artiga, S. (2022, August 22). *Covid-19 cases and deaths by race/ethnicity: Current data and changes over time.* KFF. Retrieved July 27, 2023, from www.kff.org/racial-equity-and-health-policy/issue-brief/covid-19-cases-and-deaths-by-race-ethnicity-current-data-and-changes-over-time/

Kaiser Permanente. (2023a). *About: Our model.* Retrieved August 16, 2023, from https://about.kaiserpermanente.org/commitments-and-impact/public-policy/integrated-care

Kaiser Permanente. (2023b). *What is Kaiser Permanente?* Retrieved August 16, 2023, from https://healthy.kaiserpermanente.org/learn/what-is-kaiser-permanente

Kaiser Permanente. (2023c, June 30). *Fast facts: Our company.* Retrieved August 16, 2023, from https://about.kaiserpermanente.org/who-we-are/fast-facts

Kaiser Permanente. (n.d.). *About: A workplace for all.* Retrieved August 16, 2023, from https://about.kaiserpermanente.org/commitments-and-impact/public-policy/integrated-care https://about.kaiserpermanente.org/commitments-and-impact/equity-inclusion-and-diversity/a-workplace-for-all

Medstar Health. (2023a). *About Medstar health.* Retrieved August 7, 2023, from www.medstarhealth.org/about

Medstar Health. (2023b). *Facts and figures Medstar health.* Retrieved August 7, 2023, from www.medstarhealth.org/about/facts-and-figures

Medstar Health. (2023c). *Healthcare services.* Retrieved August 7, 2023, from www.medstarhealth.org/services

Medstar Health. (2023d). *Awards and recognitions: Medstar health.* Retrieved August 7, 2023, from www.medstarhealth.org/about/medstar-health-awards-and-recognitions

Ministry of Health and Wellness (MOHW). (n.d.). *Vision for health 2030: Ten year strategic plan 2019–2030.* Retrieved August 9, 2023, from MOHW-Vision-for-Health-2030-Final.pdf

Moore, K. (2022, May 19). *Racial disparities in Washington, D.C. Covid-19 vaccine administration.* Legal Defense Fund. Retrieved July 27, 2023, from www.naacpldf.org/naacp-publications/ldf-blog/chocolate-city-vanilla-vaccine-racial-disparities-in-washington-dc-covid-19-vaccine-administration/

National Academies of Sciences, Engineering, and Medicine. (2021). *Implementing high-quality primary care: Rebuilding the foundation of health care* (L. McCauley, R. L. Phillips, Jr., M. Meisnere, & S. K. Robinson, Eds.). The National Academies Press. https://doi.org/10.17226/25983

NHS. (2019). *The NHS long term plan.* Retrieved July 27, 2023, from www.longtermplan.nhs.uk/wp-content/uploads/2019/08/nhs-long-term-plan-version-1.2.pdf

Ramos, M. C., Barreto, J. O. M., Shimizu, H. E., de Moraes, A. P. G., & da Silva, E. N. (2020). Regionalization for health improvement: A systematic review. *PLOS One,* 15(12), e0244078. https://doi.org/10.1371/journal.pone.024407

Ross University School of Medicine. (2023). *US vs. Canadian healthcare: What is the difference?* Retrieved August 5, 2023, from https://medical.rossu.edu/about/blog/us-vs-canadian-healthcare

Shi, L., & Singh, D. A. (2022). *Delivering healthcare in America: A systems approach* (8th ed.). Jones & Bartlett Learning.

Tikkanen, R., Osborn, R., Mossialos, E., Djordjevic, A., & Wharton, G. A. (2020). *International health care system profiles: Canada.* Retrieved August 5, 2023, from www.commonwealthfund.org/international-health-policy-center/countries/canada

United Kingdom National Health Service (NHS). (2021). *About the NHS.* Retrieved July 23, 2023, from www.nhs.uk/nhs-england/about-the-nhs/

United States Agency for International Development. (n.d.). *Strengthening community health systems.* Retrieved October 3, 2023, from www.usaid.gov/global-health/health-systems-innovation/health-systems/strengthening-community-health-systems

---

ANALYTICAL EXERCISE

1. You need to suggest a team to work together to plan a regional healthcare system. What kinds of professionals would you suggest to become members of this team? Give the rationale for your responses.

2. You are a member of a multidisciplinary team that is planning to create a regional healthcare system in a _____ area.

   a. What are some general considerations that the team should discuss? Give the rationale for your responses.

   b. What are some inclusion considerations that the team should discuss? Give the rationale for your responses.

CASE STUDY

You have been hired to be a member of a team to evaluate a regional healthcare system that will serve residents from a variety of backgrounds. This region in particular contains areas that are poverty stricken, and the citizens are prone to various healthcare problems related to diet, lack of exercise, and lack of access to healthcare services. Due to their socio-economic status, many of the residents in these areas do not regularly engage in preventative care. This region also has very clear socioeconomic spatial divides that are exacerbated by infrastructure like highways, railroad tracks, and waterbodies.

- Considering these challenges, what recommendations would you make to ensure the inclusive design and planning of this system's facilities?
- What considerations should the team discuss?

2

HEALTH SCIENCES CENTERS AND ACADEMIC MEDICAL CENTERS

Marianne Graffam

Introduction

Outside of residential healthcare, which includes assisted living and senior care facilities, typical healthcare spaces are divided into two broad categories: inpatient and outpatient facilities. However, with approximately 6% of the healthcare market nationwide (Burke et al., 2017), research and academic-based medical and health sciences centers and teaching hospitals have a small but impactful footprint within the national healthcare infrastructure. Academic medical centers (AMCs) consist of inpatient and outpatient medical facilities with Joint Commission accreditation. They are organizationally and administratively integrated with medical and allied health schools and are where specialized health concerns are welcomed and treated. Even though both AMCs and teaching hospitals are affiliated with a medical school, unlike AMCs, teaching hospitals do not issue medical degrees (Definitive Healthcare, 2022).

The mission of any hospital or healthcare system is to primarily provide clinical care, which is inherently different from AMCs due to their strategic

DOI: 10.4324/9781003414902-3

partnerships with teaching institutions and medical schools across the country, placing them at the intersection of education, research, and practice. In addition to providing the best possible patient care, the most significant objective of an AMC is the use of cutting-edge technologies, therapies, and resources enhanced by advanced research and education. The aim is to create environments where students, healthcare providers, and researchers can collaborate, exploring the limitless possibilities of the future of medicine, patient care, and community health. This collaborative environment fosters engagement to help improve health equity by creating systems that work together with institutional community health initiatives and partner with neighborhood groups (Association of American Medical Colleges [AAMC], 2023). Many of these initiatives are nationally recognized and are sought out for various specialties, advanced research, and practices. Two examples of this are the University of Texas MD Anderson Cancer Center and the Mayo Clinic.

Academic Medical Centers

AMCs are continuously evolving to educate and train future medical professionals. This evolution includes utilizing emerging technological and scientific advancements, conducting state-of-the-art research, and providing highly specialized clinical care services for better patient care. Due to this wide range of objectives that AMCs strive to fulfill, they commonly serve as anchors of their community because of their connection to universities and their mission to fulfill many social and economic needs of the area. Each AMC becomes a critical element to the health and vibrancy of the communities that surround them and often one of the region's major employers. Additionally, AMCs provide resources for public services and education for community members as a measure to help improve the overall economic and physical health of the region. Because of these objectives, the American Hospital Association (AHA) identifies many AMCs as Metropolitan Anchor Hospitals (Hartzman et al., 2022).

To address some of the current health and socioeconomic issues facing communities, AMCs have begun to broaden their research missions to include population health, utilizing research and community engagement to work toward improving health at multiple levels and scales. This includes the overall health of communities and the personalized medicine scale, where providers are able to use an individual's genetic profile to help guide treatment and decisions made regarding the prevention, diagnosis, and treatment of disease. This range of community outreach and personalized care has a significant impact regionally and nationally due to documentation and knowledge sharing that is innate within the makeup of AMCs.

AMCs can also help improve the health of their region by expanding their clinical missions to address wellness and social determinants of health, such as access to affordable housing or transportation, food, and employment (Health Research Institute [HRI], 2019). They often serve as safety net hospitals and trauma centers within their region. These medical centers are able to provide highly specialized clinical care and have the resources and ability to serve the most severely ill, injured, and vulnerable patients and provide care to the marginalized, uninsured, and underinsured population. In order for AMCs to continue this mission, however, they will need to establish the needed infrastructure to support long-term community partnerships, adopt policies to support continued engagement, and study new ways of integrating community members in roles as advisors and collaborators (Wilkins & Alberti, 2019).

A vital part of the success of any AMC is the rigor, depth, and range of its research programs. The ability to advance research through clinical trials and develop new possibilities in medicine, patient care, and population health can change the healthcare landscape and often have positive impacts beyond the immediate region. Positive outcomes of these clinical trials advance the practice of medicine and provide more efficient treatments and approaches that become a part of standard practice across the country. This work informs and improves current healthcare practices by creating new therapies and treatments that set the standard for care. Examples of past advances resulting from research and academic-based institutions include vaccines against pneumonia, treatments for HIV/AIDS, cancer research and treatment options, and imaging technologies such as the development of magnetic resonance imaging (MRI), to name a few.

Rigorous academic and research-based healthcare practice also fosters peer-reviewed published papers, journals, or books to share knowledge nationally and globally to advance medicine. Unusual diagnoses are also good topics for publication to gather insights from other research institutions nationwide. With research and teaching happening adjacent to each other, the primary investigators who lead clinical trials seek innovative solutions and ideas to solve complex medical problems. This way of weaving teaching and research together is essential to creating an environment where the next generation of physicians, healthcare professionals, caregivers, and primary investigators implementing research are empowered to advance current practices and scientific discoveries.

Evidence shows that there are many benefits to having an AMC within a community. Physicians and researchers tend to practice in close geographic proximity to where they trained, leading to a more robust pool of healthcare providers and better patient outcomes within a given AMC region. Multiple studies have also demonstrated better outcomes, on average, for patients treated at AMCs due to innovative practices augmented by a robust research program, showing that treatment in a market with a more significant AMC presence was associated with lower mortality and remaining healthy for a more extended period after treatment. These findings suggest that the impact of AMCs on clinical outcomes extends beyond direct patient care and that there are spillover effects of AMCs on outcomes for patients in the broader healthcare market (Burke et al., 2023).

While anyone can be admitted and treated at an AMC, it is often not the most cost-effective option for patients with typical health concerns (Torrey, 2020). The operation of an AMC is often more costly than community hospitals due to a combination of the education and research programs and providing care to the indigent patient population and therefore cannot be as efficient as a community hospital (Torrey, 2020). However, patients with rare diseases, undiagnosed symptoms, and more complex conditions would benefit the most from receiving treatment at an AMC due to their wide range of services. These patients meet the eligibility requirements for treatment at a Level 1 trauma center, where total care for every aspect of injury, from prevention to rehabilitation, can be provided. An AMC that is part of a more extensive healthcare network like University Medical Center – New Orleans (UMC-NO) can strategically utilize the various community and specialty hospitals and clinics within the larger (LCMC Health) system to serve the needs of the individual patient best while still benefiting from resources of the research and academic-based medical and health sciences center.

Historically, AMCs have offset academic and research expenses with clinical care while still providing services to the uninsured and underinsured due to their safety net hospital status. Contemporarily, however, many AMCs often feel pressure to create a better balance between care and cost. In this period of escalating healthcare expenses, the speed and cost of expanding technologies in medicine and scientific advancements and the current national focus on addressing overall population health have the most significant economic impact on AMCs. The Health Research Institute (HRI), after surveying dozens of AMC thought leaders and executives, came to the consensus that for the future success of AMCs, the approach to delivering care at various systems may need to adjust and focus their operations on highlighting their strengths in order to deliver new value to the demographic they serve (HRI, 2019). Many of those interviewed believe that the future of AMCs will be a hybrid of four distinct models: product leader, experience leader, integrator, and health manager, with each model type having a different financial constraint that the individual medical center will need to balance.

The product leaders pursue growing market shares in profitable procedures by delivering high quality and the most advanced care. Many academic medical systems and teaching hospitals often build "centers of excellence" focusing on specific diseases or conditions, such as stroke, heart, and cancers. The experience leaders target the patient experience over their lifetime so that they can attract and retain customers. They draw inspiration from customer-focused industries to tailor the patient's experience by focusing on design, marketing, and service delivery strategies. The integrator balances care and coverage to create greater consumer convenience and affordability. Health managers strive to improve and manage the health of a community over time and address the social determinants of health that are impacting patients in their market (HRI, 2019).

The Design and Planning of AMCs

The model type in which facilities deliver patient care and conduct research impacts the design approach. Buildings and spaces are among the many tools that aid healthcare providers in performing effectively. The environments that designers and medical planners create should be informed by the organization's missions and should set the foundation for healthcare providers to do their best work. Thoughtful design and meaningful integration of AMC's multifaceted missions into the built environment can impact the success of everyday practice.

Through the inclusion of and collaboration with end users, designers have the capacity to create spaces that meet the functional needs of the patients receiving care, health providers, students, and researchers. Additionally, designers can ensure that these individuals are given an environment that is comfortable and safe, enabling resourceful collaboration.

Inclusive design is vital to the future growth and success of any healthcare system, integrating the programs and mission of AMCs to help support the everyday activities of the people they serve. The spaces within AMCs serve the most vulnerable populations, and the design should aim to provide equitable, accessible, and inclusive spaces that promote the safety and health of all users. Due to the complex nature of hospitals and healthcare spaces, function and clarity in the design are essential, having a significant impact on a user's impression of the built environment. AMC programs are usually centered around the current health conditions impacting the community and the range and focus of academic practice and research. The breadth and evolving nature of academic and research components and user groups add complexity to the planning and design approach of AMCs. Designers will need to plan for current needs and future growth by incorporating flexible spaces that include universal design elements and have the ability to adapt to patient care needs with limited disruption.

Planners of new AMCs should create master plans that allow for operational efficiency, flexibility, and future expansion. For example, one can strategically anchor the perimeter of an urban site and planned green space and later expand it for additional program needs. The footprint of the various campus components can also be systematically increased by adding patient towers, inpatient hospital blocks, or an outpatient ambulatory care building in the future with minimal impact to the built structure.

There is a collaboration with Eskew Dumez Ripple and Perkins & Will for the new University of South Alabama (USA) College of Medicine, which is associated with USA Health. This collaboration is designed to implement one of the ongoing transformations of medical schools across the country. Research and medical education, often housed in separate facilities, will be combined into one building so that medical students can engage more with research and cutting-edge technologies and mirror the collaboration that happens at AMCs. Additionally, impromptu encounters that promote and encourage the exchange of new ideas and collaborations can occur between disciplines.

Conclusion

During this current period of continuous, rapid change in healthcare and higher education due to the speed of advancement in science and research, academic medical and health sciences centers are advancing the world of healthcare and how clinical care is provided at an unprecedented pace. With physicians, nurses, researchers, and teachers working in unison, patients have better access to the latest medical breakthroughs and clinical trials not available at other hospitals. AMCs' triple-focused mission and the extensive range of services needed to provide training for our next generation of healthcare providers and leaders position them to create new opportunities and solidify their place as anchor institutions in their communities. They do so by delivering high-quality, specialized care; integrating advanced technological resources, and training healthcare professionals. Additionally, they deliver healthcare while furthering cutting-edge research and addressing issues of disparities in the access and delivery of healthcare and opportunities for overall wellness. In conjunction with policy and ongoing community engagement, design has the capacity to address some of those disparities by creating spaces that enable all users a sense of safety and equity.

References

Association of American Medical Colleges. (2023). *Building a systems approach to community health and health equity for academic health centers*. Retrieved October 4, 2023, from www.aamchealthjustice.org/resources/health-equity-systems

Burke, L. G., Burke, R. C., Orav, E. J., Duggan, C. E., Figueroa, J. F., & Jha, A. K. (2023). Association of academic medical center presence with clinical outcomes at neighboring community hospitals among Medicare beneficiaries. *JAMA Network Open*, 6(2), e2254559. https//doi.org/10.1001/jamanetworkopen.2022.54559

Burke, L. G., Frakt, A. B., Khullar, D., Orav, E. J., & Jha, A. K. (2017). Association between teaching status and mortality in US Hospitals. *JAMA*, 317(20), 2105–2113. https://doi.org/10.1001/jama.2017.5702

Definitive Healthcare. (2022, December 9). *Top 25 largest academic medical centers*. Retrieved May 1, 2023, from www.definitivehc.com/resources/healthcare-insights/top-largest-academic-medical-centers

Hartzman, A., Mancino, M., Martinez, L., & Gorman, C. (2022, October). *Exploring metropolitan anchor hospitals and the communities they serve*. The American Hospital Association (AHA).

Health Research Institute. (2019). *America's future academic medical centers: Forging new identities in the new health economy*. Retrieved May 1, 2023, from www.pwc.com/us/en/industries/health-industries/health-research-institute/americas-future-academic-medical-centers.html

Torrey, T. (2020, February 27). *Pros and cons of academic hospital care.* Retrieved May 1, 2023, from www.verywellhealth.com/teaching-or-university-hospital-2614877

Wilkins, C. H., & Alberti, P. M. (2019). Shifting academic health centers from a culture of community service to community engagement and integration. *Academic Medicine: Journal of the Association of American Medical Colleges, 94*(6), 763. https://doi.org/10.1097/ACM.0000000000002711

3

HEALTHCARE IN HOSPITALS

Ronnie Ursin

Introduction

Globally, an estimated 421 million persons are hospitalized each year (World Health Organization [WHO], 2019). Hospitals provide healthcare services to diverse groups of clients across the lifespan who are sick, injured, and/or physically impaired (HMC Architects, 2019). Therefore, their design should be focused on enhancing health and quality and providing a safe environment for all who use them. Furthermore, the design of healthcare settings, such as hospitals, should be efficient, practical, and inclusive of providing an element of comfort and healing for people being served and the well-being of their employees (Wikoff, 2021; Neenan Archistruction, n.d.). Nurses are among the largest professional group in hospitals; they believe that healthcare design influences how we interact with one another, the type and level of care given and received, family involvement, the internal environment, and comfort (Zimmerman, 2011). In this chapter, the author discusses the design features that support inclusive considerations for clients, their

DOI: 10.4324/9781003414902-4

families, and staff in hospital spaces such as patient and waiting rooms, the emergency department, and the surgical suite.

Socially Inclusive Architecture

One way to promote inclusivity in hospitals is to design for *social inclusion*, that is, "looking at a broad spectrum of occupants – from the young and the old, of every diversity, across all economic lines – and what they need to feel comfortable in a space and receptive to a health interaction" (HMC Architects, 2019, para 1).

Socially inclusive architecture considers end-user preferences in their design, and according to HMC Architects (2019) it is important to:

- Ensure that there are accommodations for persons who are large in size. Accommodations such as seats that are wider than usual and extra space in rooms and bathrooms for easy movement should be made. Accommodation for different body sizes is also recommended by Tylka et al. (2014). They suggest the availability of furniture, gowns, and equipment (for example, blood pressure cuffs and scales) for different body sizes.
- Exceed the Americans with Disability Act accessibility requirements. And, of note, the World Health Organization produced seven modules and tip sheets to help guide health facilities toward adopting more disability-inclusive practices (WHO, 2020). Included in considerations for design are effective communication, access, and inclusivity.
- Promote cultural inclusivity by having multilanguage signs and ensure that there are clear, big signs for the visually impaired. Poorly designed signs have been attributed to the expansion of existing facilities, but it is important to have competent signage systems when designing and redesigning hospitals (Rodrigues et al., 2019). Loop Media (2023) suggests the benefits of digital signage in the healthcare industry. Some of these benefits include real-time updates on waiting periods, the display of educational information, and the facilitation of communication between stakeholders. Digital signage could prove effective in wayfinding, could reduce wait-time anxiety, allow for real-time messaging, and result in faster diagnosis, creating healthier staff-patient relationships

and better visibility (Loop Media). Furthermore, hospitals should consider incorporating Rodriques et al.'s (2019) nine design categories during the design and installation process of their signage systems. Their design categories are "(1) text formatting; (2) information hierarchy and density; (3) language and terminology; (4) symbols and pictograms; (5) colors; (6) placement, dimensions, and typology of signs; (7) illumination, visibility, and legibility; (8) standardization; (9) inclusivity and user characteristics" (p. 48).

- Incorporate braille and/or web-enabled applications into the building's infrastructure in consideration of the visually impaired. Patient experience can be improved by incorporating tactile signage that is strategically placed and of an appropriate size (Myerson & West, 2015).
- Ensure that there are areas for children to play in the waiting room and/or in an outside garden.
- Ensure that there are areas for therapy and service animals to wait with and for their owners and also areas where they can relieve themselves.
- Incorporate automatic doors so that clients and patrons do not have to pull hardware, and if hardware is used, ensure that it is easy to pull.
- Provide stations where mobile devices can be charged; this helps families to stay connected.
- Incorporate handrails along corridors so that they are accessible to patients, patrons, and staff.
- Provide toilet rooms that are gender neutral.

Hospital administrators should ensure that their designers collaborate with a multidisciplinary team in the design and/or redesign of their facility. The multidisciplinary team should consist of professionals and nonprofessionals who have the expertise and ability to assist with the creation of an inclusive healthcare environment. There should also be patient and family representation on the team because they are the major consumers of healthcare in the hospital.

Patient Rooms and Waiting Rooms/Areas

Patients and their families who enter hospitals spend much of their time in the patient rooms and/or waiting rooms and areas. How a space is organized and the design impact can be felt by persons who access that space

(Lamb, 2021). Therefore, this section focuses on consideration for the design of patient rooms and waiting rooms and areas.

Patient Rooms

Patient rooms such as those on medical-surgical units in hospitals constitute a significant component of a hospital building project. There is a significant need to ensure patient rooms are designed to provide comfort and are environments for healing. The staff who function and deliver care to patients in their rooms should also be considered. Lavender et al. (2020) support design features that improve the patient experience, reduce the physical and cognitive demand on staff, and improve workflows. Beenu Interior Design (2014) suggests the inclusion of features such as lighting, accessible fixtures, comfortable patient suites, and entry points designed with patient comfort and staff needs in mind.

Inclusive designs should include considerations for the entry points, bathrooms and restrooms, biohazard standards, lighting, accessibility of gloves and sanitizer, bed, windows, sleepers, televisions, whiteboard, seating area, environment control (air conditioning/heat), bathroom, and storage. Table 3.1 provides design features relevant for the design process (Lavender et al., 2020).

Table 3.1 Design Features – Patient Room

Design Features	Design Guidelines
Room door	Use an easily operated manual sliding door rather than a swing or folding door
Staff sink	Inside the room, near the door
Biohazard containers	Inside the room, near the door
In-room storage	Provide adequate space for in-room mobile medical supply storage with a horizontal work surface that can be used by staff
Bed/door/window	• Locate patient bed such that the patient can see out of the window without assuming an awkward posture • Locate patient bed such that the patient can see who is entering the room • Locate patient bed such that the patient can communicate with people in the family area

Table 3.1 (Continued)

Design Features	Design Guidelines
Television	Position the TV so that the patient can view it comfortably when sitting or lying in bed or the recliner
Visual barrier	Provide a visual barrier, such as a privacy curtain, that affords privacy from the hallway and family seating area when needed or desired
Whiteboard	Position whiteboard such that it can be easily viewed by staff and patients and easily updated by staff
Seating/bed	In addition to space for a recliner, provide space for visitor/staff seating in close proximity to the patient's bed
Wall outlets	Provide an adequate number of electrical outlets that are accessible by the patient when in bed or in the recliner
Lighting and controls	Provide the patient with control of the electric lighting, including ambient room lighting and reading light, from the bed and the recliner

Lavender et al. (2020)

Waiting Rooms and Areas

The design of waiting rooms and areas in hospitals is often influenced by budgetary constraints, and these spaces can reflect health inequities (Lamb, 2021). While the management of care is critical, the design of considerate healthcare spaces can influence not only the patient experience but also the experience for their families. Terry (2019) suggests key areas for the improvement of waiting rooms, which directly impact the overall patient experience; these key areas include safe accommodation, comfort, and welcoming amenities. Lamb (2021) includes flooring as an element of design in this space. Safe accommodations, comfort, and welcoming amenities include concepts such as chair design and size, seating arrangements, infection control, textiles and surface material, cleaning, refreshments, and reading materials (Terry, 2019). Table 3.2 depicts considerations for the design of inclusive waiting rooms (Terry, 2019; Michael Graves Architecture and Design, 2023).

Table 3.2 Design Features – Waiting Room

Concepts	Descriptors
Chairs	Higher weight capacity Flexible vertical seat adjustment Comfort (cushion) Large handles and armrests Table arm with pull-up tables Facilitate sitting and standing
Seating arrangements	Cluster seating vs ganged seating Quiet areas for noise control Line of sight (reception and doorway)
Accessibility	Wide aisles Power ports for electronics Easy-to-access and -operate lighting controls
Infection control	Separate areas for sick vs well patients Curated patient paths through facilities
Textile and surface	Resistant to liquid and air Ease of cleaning over time
Indoor and outdoor views	Natural lighting with complements such as lamps Artwork (soft, soothing colors)
Flooring	Carpet for noise reduction

In addition to patient rooms and waiting rooms and areas, inclusive and innovative design considerations should be applied in the emergency department and surgical suite of hospitals. These spaces warrant consideration because they are highly specialized areas within hospitals.

The Emergency Department

An emergency department (ED) is a healthcare space within a hospital facility that provides unscheduled services to patients whose conditions require immediate care. Scheduling of some healthcare services provided in EDs have occurred subsequent to changes in emergency care models. In some cases, changes have resulted in services requiring scheduling. The scope of services range from medication refill requests, to minor illnesses such as bumps and bruises, to significant trauma. The number and type of services provided depend on the size, scope, location, and availability of specialty services offered by the hospital. The definition of what makes a hospital small, medium, or large can vary, but generally, small hospitals contain fewer than 100 beds, medium hospitals contain between 100 and 499 beds, and large hospitals contain at least 500 or more beds (Gallagher Healthcare, 2018). Other factors for this definition may include whether the facility is community based, rural, or urban (American Hospital Association, 2023). All EDs tend to have general features, but size determines the number of available beds and the design of the layout.

Design Considerations

In 2018, Walid Tarawneh provided perspective on the main considerations in the design and planning of an ED, indicating ED design is influenced by the needs of patients, staff requirements, and the characteristics of emergency medicine. Design considerations for EDs should include needs of patients, staffing, clinical services, temperature, lighting, location (on/off campus), and size (Tarawneh, 2018). Functionality between all aspects of the ED must be considered, including movement between patient waiting areas, triage, staff workspaces, decontamination spaces, reception, and ambulance entry points.

The ambulance entry point is a vital aspect of emergency services. The design of ambulance entry points, how vehicles access them, and provisions for the number of ambulances allowed for the safe transport of patients should be considered (March, n.d.). Ambulances should have direct access to the entry doors. Ambulance pathways should not have physical barriers and should be easily accessible from the roads and adjacent parking lots. The disembarkation of patients should be obstacle-free, allowing for quick and easy access to the building/ED and easy departure from the healthcare delivery space. Design features should also include considerations for ambulance design and engineering issues and requirements for the urgent, discrete cleaning of ambulances. Tarawneh (2018) concludes by suggesting the inclusion of a route for relatives arriving with ambulances and signage directing visitors toward ED registration and/or waiting areas.

Security Services

Security services have become a significant part of the design of EDs. One of the responsibilities of security personnel should be to control the activities in the space and maintain an access-free ambulance bay. These services are usually posted at the entrances of EDs. This is particularly so as the volume of patients entering hospitals via EDs increases and security concerns rise. Designs need to consider adequate, visible, and functional spaces for security personnel. Many ambulance security desks are sized to also allow for police officers. Some EDs have established police substations within them (March, n.d.).

Patient Access

Exterior features should complement emergency rooms, considering access for patients who arrive at the ED by other modes of transportation, through private transport, and via ambulant means (March, n.d.; Tarawneh, 2018). In this situation, entry points should be clearly delineated and separate from the ambulance entry. This design approach is to protect patient privacy. The entrance to the ED should not be used for general purposes such as pass-through access to the hospital by staff and nonemergency patients. Patients arriving by car may require a wheelchair; therefore, the design should include an adjacent structure that supports transfer from a vehicle and direct access to the entrance of a facility. The access needs of young children and their caregivers/guardians are similar to those of persons with disabilities. Parking spaces should be allocated for families with these situations during design planning, allowing for easy access to the ED.

The Surgical Suite

The surgical suite is an important space in hospitals. There are numerous considerations to contemplate when designing a safe, effective, and efficient surgical suite. Advances in medical practice have forced changes in the design of surgical suites. Unified suite designs have evolved to occupy more than 500 square feet of space, creating capacity for multifunctional use, and grouped surgical suites with a core functional space (Avante Medical Surgical, 2017). Healthcare design is also influenced by the types of care provided and innovations in surgical procedures. Trends indicate that the use of minimally invasive procedures and robotics often requires larger surgical spaces. Advances in intraoperative magnetic resonance imaging (MRI) are expected to drive the demand for highly technological surgical spaces.

While the advances in surgical technology are driving the evolution of surgical space design, there are fundamental design aspects necessary for performing safe, comforting, and efficient surgical procedures. These design considerations include the size of surgical suites, as well as the location of support spaces and supply areas. Additionally, specialized surgical suites, such as hybrid operating rooms, support challenges presented during equipment integration and should be designed for patient flow, radiation safety, and workflow requirements (Steris Healthcare, 2023).

On average, a surgical suite is approximately 600 square feet (Avante Medical Surgical, 2017; Steris Healthcare, 2023). Avante expresses the necessity to build a surgical suite with longevity by considering the integration of newer technologies including endovascular, MRI, and imaging equipment. This is subsequent to the impact that innovation is having on the evolution of the surgical suite to hybrid suites; more advanced spaces may ultimately become the standard. The design size must consider equipment needs such as anesthesia machines and carts, airway carts and materials, robotic surgery, computers, large monitors, mounted ceiling booms, and mobile surgical tables. A central design theme for the surgical suite is to place the operating table at the core of the suite with support spaces arranged around it according to surgical processes.

Sterile Processing

The sterilization of equipment is required for surgical procedures taking place in operating rooms. There are specific requirements necessary for the promotion of patient and staff safety. This includes ensuring all equipment is properly sterilized and cleaned. The design of spaces where sterilization of equipment occurs should be in alignment with industry standards. Such standards are published by organizations such as The Joint Commission, Association for the Advancement of Medical Instrumentation, Association of periOperative Nurses (AORN), and the Society of Gastroenterology Nurses. Design considerations that support safe, efficient, and sterile processing spaces include location, standards, and boundaries in workflow (Owens & Minor, 2023). Guiffrida-Levesque (2021) suggests the importance of specialized finishes for decontamination and a smart dumbwaiter.

The location of a sterile processing department (SPD) plays a critical role in creating a workflow that allows for the effective turnover, management, and delivery of sterile instruments to the surgical suite (Owens & Minor, 2023). Since more than 75% of sterilized instruments are needed for surgery, positioning the department on the same floor as the surgical suite is ideal. Benefits of having the SPD and the surgical suite on the same floor include reduced time for equipment and supply delivery and the minimization of travel time through other areas of the hospital (Owens & Minor, 2023).

The decontamination room, also known as the "dirty" room, may require finishes that can withstand the movement and impact of dirty carts and the constant use of water within the space. Poured urethane resin epoxy flooring finishes are often selected due to the durability and resistance to harsh chemicals and nonslip textures (Allegheny Installations, n.d.). In addition, diamond plate wall protection made of metals like aluminum or with medium-density polyethylene are ideal for shielding walls from damage from carts and equipment. Epoxy paint or fiber-reinforced polymer (FRP) panels are often used on walls to provide an easily cleanable surface.

Agencies responsible for regulatory standards and guidelines in sterile processing have effectively impacted designs for years. According to Brooks and Reimer (2019), the standards, regulations, and recommendations are changing daily as sterile processing and operating room associates try to balance modifications in process with meeting the expectations of daily operations. Two regulatory bodies that influence sterile processing guidelines and design standards are The Joint Commission and Centers for Medicare and Medicaid. Both organizations set rigorous standards for patient safety and improving health outcomes, but their methods may vary across the healthcare sector. A standard practice with the design of an SPD is to provide clear demarcations between soiled, clean, and sterile instruments with the placement of physical barriers. An effective workflow will allow for the streamlined movement of soiled instruments through decontamination to their place in the next surgical kit, ensuring all SPD staff have the space to move freely and preventing the need for them to enter sterile spaces unnecessarily (Brooks & Reimer, 2019). These considerations are vital when planning and designing an SPD that maximizes workflow efficiency and space, to the benefit of all involved.

Conclusion

Inclusive design of hospitals is critical for the effective, efficient, and safe delivery of care to patients and staff directly and indirectly involved in providing their care. The design of healthcare spaces impact healthcare outcomes and experience. The focus of this chapter was on considerations for general inclusive design and design features of patient rooms, waiting rooms and areas, EDs, and surgical suites. Hospital administrators can apply these considerations in the design of other areas of the hospital with the assistance of a multidisciplinary team. Involving and engaging the end user (patients and their families) in all phases of hospital design is crucial.

References

Allegheny Installations. (n.d.). *Urethane flooring.* Retrieved July 25, 2023, from https://alleghenyinstallations.com/urethane.php#:~:text=Urethane%20floors%20are%20low%20maintenance,urethane%20material%20furnished%20and%20installed

American Hospital Association. (2023). *Fast facts on U.S. hospitals, 2023.* Retrieved July 25, 2023, from www.aha.org/statistics/fast-facts-us-hospitals

Avante Medical Surgical. (2017). *An introduction to operating room design.* Retrieved July 25, 2023, from www.dremed.com/medical_equipment_news/a-basic-guide-to-setting-up-todays-or

Beenu Interior Design. (2014). *Healthcare design.* Retrieved July 25, 2023, from https://beenuinteriordesign.com/healthcare-design/#:~:text=Healthcare%20Design%20is%20focused%20on,and%20staff%20needs%20in%20mind

Brooks, A., & Reimer, J. (2019). Surveying sterile processing and how regulatory bodies have shaped the sterile processing community. *Infection Control Today.* www.infectioncontroltoday.com/view/surveying-sterile-processing-and-how-regulatory-bodies-have-shaped-sterile

Gallagher Healthcare. (2018). *What are the different types of hospitals?* Retrieved July 25, 2023, from www.gallaghermalpractice.com/blog/post/what-are-the-different-types-of-hospitals/#:~:text=There%20are%20three%20primary%20classifications,hospitals%3A%20500%20or%20more%20beds

Guiffrida-Levesque, A. (2021). *Planning & designing a central sterile processing department.* Retrieved July 25, 2023, from www.linkedin.com/pulse/planning-designing-central-sterile-processing-annette/

HMC Architects. (2019). *Adaptive spaces: The need for socially inclusive architecture in healthcare.* Retrieved November 17, 2023, from https://hmcarchitects.com/news/adaptive-spaces-the-need-for-socially-inclusive-architecture-in-healthcare-2019-07-24/

Lamb, M. (2021). Health inequity by design: Waiting rooms and patient stress. *Frontier Communication, 6,* 6–10. www.frontiersin.org/articles/10.3389/fcomm.2021.667381/full

Lavender, S., Sommerich, C., Sanders, E., Evans, K. D., Li, J., Radin Umar, R. Z., & Patterson, E. S. (2020). Developing evidence-based design guidelines for medical/surgical hospital patient rooms that meet the needs of staff, patients, and visitors. *HERD, 13*(1). https://doi.org/10.1177/1937586719856009

Loop Media. (2023). *The benefits of digital signage in healthcare.* Retrieved July 25, 2023, from www.linkedin.com/pulse/benefits-digital-signage-healthcare-loopforbusiness/

March, J. H. (n.d.). Design considerations for a safer emergency department. *American College of Emergency Physicians.* www.acep.org/siteassets/sites/acep/media/safety-in-the-ed/designconsiderationsforsaferemergencydepartment.pdf

MAS in Collective Housing. (2023). *Architectural design: Definition, types, and examples.* Retrieved July 25, 2023, from www.mchmaster.com/news/architectural-design-definition-types-and-examples/#:~:text=Architectural%20design%20is%20a%20discipline,certain%20tools%20and%20especially%2C%20creativity

Michael Graves Architecture and Design. (2023). *Patient room furniture.* Retrieved July 25, 2023, from www.michaelgraves.com/projects/patient-room-furniture

Myerson, J., & West, J. (2015, November 12–13). *Make it better: How universal design principles can have an impact on healthcare services to improve the patient experience.* Proceedings of the Universal Design in Education Conference; Dublin, Ireland. https://arrow.tudublin.ie/cgi/viewcontent.cgi?article=1005&context=exdesthe1

Neenan Archistruction. (n.d.). *The importance of design in healthcare buildings.* Retrieved July 25, 2023, from www.neenan.com/the-importance-of-design-in-healthcare-buildings/#:~:text=Better%20Design%20Means%20Better%20Patient%20Care&text=This%20is%20because%20a%20well,%2C%20family%20members%2C%20and%20staff

Owens & Minor. (2023). *3 design considerations for sterile processing departments.* Retrieved July 25, 2023, from www.halyardhealth.com/articles/sterilization/3-design-considerations-for-sterile-processing-departments

Rodrigues, R., Coelho, R., & Tavares, J. M. R. S. (2019). Healthcare signage design: A review on recommendations for effective signing. *HERD: Health Environment Research and Design Journal, 12*(3), 45–65. https://doi.org/10.1177/1937586718814822

Steris Healthcare. (2023). *What is a hybrid operating room?* Retrieved July 25, 2023, from www.steris.com/healthcare/knowledge-center/surgical-equipment/what-is-a-hybrid-operating-room#:~:text=The%20average%20size%20of%20a,is%20roughly%20600%20square%20feet

Tarawneh, W. (2018). *Main considerations in design and planning of emergency department (ED) part 1.* Retrieved July 25, 2023, from www.linkedin.com/pulse/main-considerations-design-planning-emergency-ed-part-tarawneh/

Terry, J. (2019). Three ways waiting room design can transform the patient experience. *Healthcare Facilities Today.* www.healthcarefacilitiestoday.com/posts/Three-ways-waiting-room-design-can-transform-the-patient-experience-20646

Tylka, T. L., Annunziato, R. A., Burgard, D., Daníelsdóttir, S., Shuman, E., Davis, C., & Calogero, R. M. (2014). The weight-inclusive versus weight-normative approach to health: Evaluating the evidence for prioritizing well-being over weight loss. *Journal of Obesity, 2014,* 1–18. https://doi.org/10.1155/2014/983495

Wikoff, M. (2021). *5 reasons why healthcare design matters.* Retrieved July 25, 2023, from https://wikoffdesignstudio.com/5-reasons-why-healthcare-design-matters/#:~:text=Healthcare%20Design%20Influences%20Patient%20Healing&text=Healthcare%20Design%20plays%20an%20important,will%20facilitate%20the%20healing%20process

World Health Organization. (2019, March 9). *Patient safety.* Retrieved November 17, 2023, from www.who.int/news-room/facts-in-pictures/detail/patient-safety

World Health Organization. (2020). *World Health Organization disability-inclusive health services toolkit: A resource for health facilities in the Western Pacific region.* https://apps.who.int/iris/bitstream/handle/10665/336857/9789290618928-eng.pdf?sequence=1&isAllowed=y

Zimmerman, R. (2011). *Why shared hospital rooms are becoming obsolete.* Retrieved July 25, 2023, from www.wbur.org/news/2011/09/16/shared-hospital-rooms-disappearing

4

NEIGHBORHOOD, AMBULATORY SETTINGS, BIRTH CENTERS, AND MOBILE HEALTHCARE SETTINGS AND UNITS

Jessica McCarthy

Introduction

Health disparities include avoidable differences in opportunities to attain optimal health experienced by communities (Centers for Disease Control and Prevention [CDC], 2017). Community members from across the country voiced they were not able to schedule a healthcare appointment or could only schedule a healthcare appointment sometimes – this increased over 45% from 2017 to 2021 according to the Agency for Healthcare Research and Quality (AHRQ). One measure to address health disparities is to focus on the access of healthcare within our communities. This chapter will give an overview of how healthcare can be administered at a neighborhood scale.

Neighborhoods are areas where people interact and reside and are defined by geography. It is within neighborhoods where communities are formed. Communities emerge as a group of people who may have diverse

DOI: 10.4324/9781003414902-5

characteristics but are linked by shared social identity, share common perspectives, and engage in joint action in geographical locations (Haldane et al., 2019). The context of a community is identified as a significant determinant of health outcomes (Marmot et al., 1995). Every community has differing needs for health promotion and improved healthcare/outcomes. Thus, collaborative efforts with community members are essential to identify specific community needs rather than speculating about what is needed.

The initial step to address and improve healthcare in any community is to conduct a community health assessment (CHA) (Centers for Disease Control and Prevention [CDC], 2022). A CHA refers to a local, tribal, or territorial health assessment identifying vital health needs and concerns through systematic, comprehensive data collection and analysis (see Table 4.1). A CHA provides comprehensive information about the community's current health status, needs, and issues. The assessment is a proactive, comprehensive, and diverse engagement to improve results within the community. This information can help develop a tailored community health improvement plan by justifying how and where resources should be allocated to best meet community needs (CDC, 2022).

Table 4.1 Community Health Assessment Steps and Processes

Steps	Processes
One	Assess community through windshield survey, resident and leader interviews, and data collection
Two	Analyze and interpret data
Three	Identify needs and concerns within community
Four	Prioritize needs: include community members for input
Five	Develop action plan: include evidence-based interventions and support of innovative practices
Six	Implement action plan
Seven	Evaluate and revise plan as needed

Adapted from CDC (2022). *Public health professionals gateway community health assessments & health improvement plans*. Retrieved September 2, 2023, from www.cdc.gov/publichealthgateway/cha/plan.html

It is important to incorporate multisector collaborations in a community assessment to support joint ownership in addressing community needs. Assessment processes should include full transparency to advance community engagement and accountability. The assessment phase must incorporate the use of the highest-quality data pooled from diverse public and private sources.

A community health improvement plan (CHIP) should be developed after the completion of the CHA. This plan will address public health problems based on the results of the community health assessment. To begin, the assessment data should be analyzed and interpreted to identify the community's needs. Prioritizing the community needs is developed with feedback from the community. Once the prioritized needs are identified, the team should transition to the planning phase. When developing the plan, it is essential to incorporate evidence-based interventions and support of innovative practices. The implementation phase will put the plan into action. The final stage will be the evaluation of the plan. The strategies developed and implemented are usually updated every three to five years but may be conducted sooner if needed. The Centers for Disease Control and Prevention (CDC) has a great module and detailed guidelines for conducting a community needs assessment.

Utilizing the CHA and the CHIP within communities will improve organizational and community coordination and collaboration to address healthcare needs. Development of a trusting relationship with community members is essential throughout this process to ensure success. Establishing trust is vital, since research reveals a higher mistrust of government and organizations among rural communities and mistrust of health services among racial and ethnic minority populations in rural areas (CDC, 2022). Working with a community through the assessment, planning, implementation, and evaluation phases to address health needs will increase community members' buy-in of the process and utilization of services offered.

Meeting Healthcare Needs of Communities Post-Assessment

Each community is unique, and their needs assessment will reveal their specific healthcare needs. It is essential to identify these needs prior to beginning any type of healthcare service. In addition, the needs assessment should include a continuous evaluation process to ensure the needs are being addressed, since communities continue to evolve and change. Even though each community is different, some healthcare needs have been identified frequently within communities.

Medical Clinics

Medical clinics are a vital part of communities and are commonly viewed as the hub/coordinator for patient care. However, patients who reside in remote areas are commonly faced with obstacles in seeking care from medical clinics. Some of the social vulnerabilities experienced in these areas include housing, transportation, socioeconomic status, race, and ethnicity (Gavidia, 2021). These vulnerabilities can directly impact neighborhood access to healthcare services. In fact, these vulnerabilities impact the 172% increase in the rural-urban U.S. mortality rate from 1999 to 2019 reported by the AHRQ.

Clinics within communities will promote a sound provider-patient relationship and improve continuity of care, which has demonstrated a reduction in community mortality rates (Baker et al., 2020). It is essential to rethink how medical services and community needs are addressed. Rural areas may not have a population that can attract providers within those areas of need. However, there are measures to consider attracting healthcare providers to these areas.

A one-stop-shop facility for these rural areas is an option to be considered. Housing multiple services within one medical suite can address multiple needs for residents. The incorporation of services such as family practice, surgery, dietary services, mental health services, gym, etc., can be housed under one roof, improving access and decreasing travel time. In addition, this can disperse overhead expenses for healthcare providers. While rural areas may not be able to recruit specialists such as a mental health provider full-time, telemedicine within this office can provide access and care when needed. It is well-documented in rural communities that some residents do have concerns with confidentiality and fear or embarrassment to seek services (CDC, 2022). With a carefully constructed office, it is possible to shield what services individuals are seeking, thus increasing trust and decreasing hesitancy to seek care.

Outpatient Hospital Services

Planners, designers, and healthcare administrators should assess and evaluate the need for outpatient services before including them in neighborhoods. These services can include x-rays, laboratory tests, minor surgeries, magnetic resonance imaging (MRI), computerized tomography (CT) scans, and preventive services such as colonoscopies and mammograms. These types of hospital services can be incorporated within a medical clinic if identified as a community need. While overhead costs of equipment may be of concern, one can consider options of equipment rental, lease, contracting with nearby hospitals, and even incorporating mobile health care to serve neighborhoods as needed. Now from a labor standpoint one may consider investing in training local residents to work within the facility and also possibly cross-train workers to improve efficiency. Investing in local residents within the office can improve trust within the community and provide feedback on measures to improve provider/patient relationships (Chipp et al., 2008). While employment of community members can improve trust, it will also contribute to employment and earnings within the community as well.

Surgery Centers

Due to limited resources and few healthcare professionals in remote areas, a small-scale surgery center can be incorporated within a shared medical suite with other services. Surgery technology has grown tremendously over the past decade. Telesurgery is an emerging surgical tool that utilizes robotic technology and wireless networking to connect patients and surgeons who are geographically distant. Telesurgery overcomes limitations of geographically inaccessible surgical care, shortages of surgeons, logistical limitations of schedules, financial costs, and travel. This technology is beneficial to the patients and surgeons, providing technical accuracy and improving safety of procedures (Oki et al., 2023).

In community areas where healthcare access is limited and surgical procedures are in demand, a general surgeon may be the best fit. General surgeons are trained to diagnose and manage diseases and disorders that may require surgical procedures and can complement any remote surgeries clients may need. Surgeons as a group in remote areas enjoy the close-knit community and the lifelong kinship they endure with their patients and families (Borgstrom et al., 2022). The surgeon's doctor-patient relationship grows even stronger in these areas by providing a variety of lifesaving and elective services to many generations within the same family (Borgstrom et al., 2022).

Despite benefits for a community and a surgeon, attracting surgeons to the community may be difficult. For example, shortages persist for surgeons in small and rural communities, with only 4.2 surgeons per 100,000 compared to 6.9 in urban areas (Cohen et al., 2021). One must consider investing in community residents interested in pursuing medical training with a commitment to return home to serve their community. In addition, general surgeons can incorporate consulting surgeons through telementoring for collaboration with other specialists. Telementoring is safe and feasible (Singh et al., 2016). This is a subgroup of telemedicine in which an expert physician guides another at a different geographical site. For example, it would allow community surgeons with no formal advanced laparoscopic training to benefit from expert intraoperative advice during the performance of advanced laparoscopic procedures. It may also reduce healthcare costs by avoiding the need to refer and transfer patients to tertiary care centers (Sebajang et al., 2005).

Kidney Care and Dialysis Centers

Again, with a vision of a one-stop-shop, a community's kidney care and dialysis services can be housed within a medical clinic office and overseen by a nephrologist who can incorporate remote care when needed. One must first consider the risk factors of rural patients with kidney damage or failure and their treatment options. According to the United States Renal Data System (2018), kidney failure is greater in men versus women, but women have a greater prevalence of chronic kidney disease (see Table 4.2). In addition, racial disparities are evident when looking at those with renal failure (Shakhnoza, 2022)

When kidney damage progresses to permanent renal failure, the only options for a patient are long-term dialysis or a kidney transplant (KT). Research reveals a patient's social support, understanding, and age were the most common factors regarded by nephrologists as important in not referring patients for KT evaluation (Bartolomeo et al., 2019). Frequent, intensive,

Table 4.2 Kidney Disease Statistics

Chronic Kidney Disease		End-Stage Renal Disease	
Demographics	Statistics	Demographics	Likely to Develop
Gender • Men • Women	 12% 14%	Gender Men:Women	 Men = 1.6 times > Women
Race • Non-Hispanic Black • Hispanic • Non-Hispanic White • Non-Hispanic Asian	 16% 14% 13% 13%	Race compared to Whites Non-Hispanic Black Hispanic Non-Hispanic Asian	 4 times > Whites 2 times > Whites 2 times > Whites
Age • 65 yo and greater • 45–64 yo • 18–44 yo	 38% 12% 6%		

Adapted from U.S. Department of Health and Human Services/Centers for Disease Control and Prevention. (2021). *Chronic kidney disease in the United States, 2021.* Retrieved November 8, 2023, from www.cdc.gov/kidneydisease/publications-resources/CKD-national-facts.html%20; National Institute of Diabetes and Digestive and Kidney Diseases, National Institutes of Health/ US Department of Health and Human Services. (2022). *United States renal data system. 2022 USRDS annual data report: Epidemiology of kidney disease in the United States.* Retrieved September 22, 2023, from https://usrds-adr.niddk.nih.gov/2022.

and tailored educational programs are needed to improve waitlisting for KT, regardless of geographic location. Patients frequently withdraw from pre-KT workup due to fear of the transplant, preconceived beliefs that they will fail the workup for transplant, and financial reasons, all of which could be potentially alleviated with proper education (Bartolomeo et al., 2019).

Prevention, early treatment, and education are keys to address and decrease rates of kidney damage and failure. Identifying those at risk and addressing these issues at the community healthcare level are essential. Some of the major causes of chronic renal failure include kidney damage due to chronic diseases.

Table 4.3 Chronic Kidney Disease – Risk Factors

Risk Factors
Diabetes (common cause)
Hypertension (common cause)
Heart disease
Obesity
Family history of chronic kidney disease
Inherited kidney disorders
Past damage to the kidneys
Older age

Adapted from Shakhnoza, I., & Asalya, A. (2022). Prevention measures of chronic renal failure in adults. *Central Asian Journal of Medical and Natural Science*, 3(4), 87–89. https://cajmns.central asianstudies.org/index.php/CAJMNS/article/view/95

Birth Centers

Birth centers are facilities where prenatal (during pregnancy) care, labor and birth, and postpartum (after delivery) care are provided using midwifery and wellness models of care (Jolles et al., 2020). These centers are needed to promote the health and well-being of the mother and unborn before birth, during labor, and after birth. A birth center is freestanding, meaning it is outside of the hospital setting. Birth centers are integrated into a larger healthcare system, and midwives provide services in birth centers that transfer to higher levels of care when needed (Dubay et al., 2020).

Childbearing families cared for within this model of care attained high-quality outcomes across all geographic settings, meeting or exceeding national benchmarks (Jolles et al., 2020). The birth center model of care has established its role as a resilient model to deliver high-quality healthcare (Dubay et al., 2020). Research reveals most rural families prefer to give birth in their community, regardless of access to appropriate levels of care (Clesse et al., 2018). The system needs to be designed as an integrated, fluid system wherein communities have access to basic care, including the birth center model of care as a normative entry point (National Academies of Sciences, Engineering, and Medicine, 2020)

Table 4.4 3 Cs to Establishing Trust and Examples

3 Cs	Methods to Establish Trust	Examples
Competence	Can be automatic Can be established with leadership role	Physician with certification and degree hanging on a wall
Character	Demonstrated through behaviors	Demonstrating integrity, humility, courage, fairness, respect, inclusion, wisdom
Consistency	Seen in what is being done	Visualized and linked to others knowing the individual

Adapted from Cultural Intelligence (2020). The 3 Cs of trust. *Cultural Synergies*. https://culturalsynergies.com/the-3-cs-of-trust/#:~:text=I%20believe%20there%20are%20three,your%20investors%20and%20your%20community

Research supports the inclusion of birth centers in rural areas. One study conducted in Guatemala revealed almost half of delivery complications were successfully resolved within the birth center, and those unresolved were referred to a higher level of care (Olivas et al., 2023). Staff of a birth center must proactively prepare pregnant women to accept a referral by addressing their concerns, fears, and other barriers during prenatal classes, with hopes of preparation if a complication would occur. In addition, addressing the women's negative perceptions of hospital care and fear of mistreatment is necessary. If a referral to a higher-level of care is required, the woman's designated support person, the patient, and family were given reasons for transfer in their native language (Olivas et al., 2023). If the patient rejects the transfer, consideration to call upon community leaders to speak with the family, if time permits, is recommended. Research findings demonstrate that the major factors underlying a family's rejection of referrals include financial constraints, fear of disrespectful treatment at the higher-level facility, fear of leaving a familiar place, cultural traditions, the mothers' lack of decision-making autonomy, and the devaluation of the mothers' lives (Olivas et al., 2023). Thus, the establishment of community trust is essential.

Telehealth

Telehealth offers a multitude of solutions to the challenges of healthcare access and benefits patients, providers, and the entire community. The telehealth benefits for patients are extensive. The utilization of this service will increase access to specialists to manage and treat chronic conditions. Telehealth can provide access to health and wellness programs such as smoking cessation, nutrition, and weight loss. In addition, access to mental health services is increased with telehealth (Natafgi et al., 2018). Fewer hospitalizations and visits to the emergency room can be attributed to telehealth services (Parker et al., 2018).

Telehealth provides numerous benefits for providers. This service can increase provider-to-provider partnerships with larger healthcare institutions and universities. Access to remote patient monitoring for patients with chronic conditions such as diabetes and heart disease can be conducted by specialists and coordinated with local providers. Providers can decrease their feelings of isolation in remote areas utilizing telehealth services as well. In addition, telehealth can increase providers' access to training and continuing education (Parker et al., 2018).

Personal and healthcare expenses can be issues affecting access or the ability to provide care within some communities. The financial benefits of telehealth include decreased time off for patients to seek care from a healthcare provider. In addition, telehealth eliminates the need for childcare for both the patient and provider. Fewer in-person visits decrease expenses for patients and providers alike. Providers can have a reduction in staffing and overhead costs with telehealth. In addition, telehealth can offer an extra income stream for providers. Telehealth will allow more attention on routine and preventative health to decrease risks of the costliest health complications (Parker et al., 2018).

Telehealth Modalities

Video chat may be the most used method of telehealth, but there are several other ways to provide care to patients. This can be especially helpful in remote regions. Other telehealth options include phone calls, remote patient monitoring, secure messaging through a patient portal, and patient-to-provider or provider-to-provider video chats from smaller, local clinics or community centers (Natafgi et al., 2018).

Telehealth is especially crucial to providing health equity in remote communities. There are many ways that telehealth provides a necessary, potentially even lifesaving, lifeline for underserved patients living in remote areas.

Table 4.5 Telehealth Types

Type	Means of Communication
Video chat	Audio and video face-to-face live visits with one or more persons
Phone calls	Audio-only visit
Remote patient monitoring	Utilizes technology to engage with patients
Messaging through a patient portal	Ability to provide text messages via a secured portal

Adapted from Health Resources and Services Administration (2022). *Get started with rural telehealth: Telehealth for rural areas.* https://telehealth.hhs.gov/providers/best-practice-guides/telehealth-for-rural-areas/getting-started

Providers can offer specialty care directly to patients or consult with healthcare providers for conditions that disproportionately affect underserved patient populations. Patients of color can use telehealth to connect with providers that make them feel more comfortable and safer. Telehealth also offers more access to translation services for non-English speakers. Assistive technology can be made available over telehealth to patients with visual, hearing, or cognitive impairments. LGBTQ+ telehealth providers can prescribe necessary treatments, including mental health counseling, gender-affirming hormones, and HIV/AIDS prevention and treatment (Health Resources and Services Administration, 2022).

Results from a recent systematic literature review suggest satisfaction with the use of eHealth and telehealth tools was generally positive across the various studies examined (Parker et al., 2018). However, the sole reliance on electronic tools to deliver health services may not enhance a patient's ability to obtain, process, and understand relevant health information. As such, telediagnosis services that only focus on access issues and ignore how individuals in vulnerable populations process and understand the information shared may exacerbate existing health disparities (Parker et al., 2018).

Several forms of telehealth technologies are commonly in use currently. Video conferencing is a system that allows two or more people/locations to communicate using simultaneous two-way audio and video transmissions (Parker et al., 2018). Systems often utilize low-cost, high-capacity broadband telecommunication services and, by using video compression techniques, allow for lifelike face-to-face interactions. Store-and forward data, images, or videos utilize a technique of capturing and transmitting information in formats such as video, photograph, x-ray images, high-resolution dermatology images, text reports, etc., to an intermediate location, which sends the information to another intermediate or final station at a time in the future (Parker et al., 2018). This system is useful in those situations where real-time communication is not necessary, and the reviewer reads batches of files/ studies at their discretion. Examples include tele-dermatology, cardiology electrocardiogram (EKG) readings, radiology study interpretations, and pulmonary function test readings by pulmonologists (Parker et al., 2018).

Remote patient monitoring is a type of ambulatory healthcare option that allows a patient to use a mobile medical device to perform routine testing and send the data to their healthcare team in real time (Parker et al., 2018). The devices can be in the patient's home or other location in addition to a healthcare or chronic care facility. Examples include diabetes monitors, heart and blood pressure monitors, and tele–intensive care unit (ICU) monitoring (Natafgi et al., 2018). Mobile health or mHealth/home health care is a general term for mobile phone or wireless technology used in medical care, often used in the context of expanding services to the developing world but not exclusive to the mission of the emergency department (Lukens, 2016). In special circumstances, such as disaster management or austere health conditions, telehealth services provide help for episodic needs and use a few wired, wireless, radio, and satellite communication methods to enable healthcare to be provided when other means may not be feasible or practical (Lukens, 2016). Telemedicine has the potential to reduce the number of transfers of emergency department patients and generate some revenue for rural facilities despite associated technology costs, while incurring substantial patient savings (Natafgi et al., 2018).

Home Health Services

Patients access a medical clinic to receive care and services needed, while telehealth can be utilized if a person-to-person visit is not possible or not needed. However, there are times when patients in various geographic locations, for example, rural areas, require personal care but are not able to physically go to the facility. Home health visits provide an option for individuals who are homebound and require medical care. These services can be offered to complement services provided within a medical clinic in rural areas. Home health services can allow healthcare providers to care for individuals within their home environment. This allows an opportunity for providers to assess their home for safety issues, perform risk assessments, and evaluate other things that may be needed for the patient.

Conclusion

All neighborhoods need equitable access to healthcare. Research revealed remote areas identify access to healthcare as the single most important factor in terms of health priorities among communities (Bolin et al., 2015). Addressing the needs of patients within a community must be individualized. Also, one must recognize the community's culture and ensure it is respected and incorporated when caring for patients. Each community will have individualized needs and expectations of healthcare. Research supports collaboration with community members for improving community health can be very effective (MacQueen et al., 2001). While many services, as discussed, are available for neighborhoods, ensuring services are accessible to all should be a priority. Our neighborhood communities are where prevention and intervention take place (MacQueen et al., 2001). It is here we can make a difference, promoting health through prevention, early detection, treatments to reduce chronic disease and complications and providing services where there are complications in an individual's health.

References

Agency for Healthcare Research and Quality. (n.d.). *Ability to schedule a routine appointment among adults, number of people in thousands, United States, 2002 to 2021.* Medical Expenditure Panel. Retrieved September 2, 2023, from https://datatools.ahrq.gov/meps-hc?tab=accessibility-and-quality-of-care&dash=16

Baker, R., Freeman, G., Haggerty, J., Bankart, M., & Nockels, K. (2020). Primary medical care continuity and patient mortality: A systematic review. *British Journal of General Practice, 70*(698), e600–e611. https://doi.org/10.3399/bjgp20X71228

Bartolomeo, K., Gandhir, A., Lipinski, M., Romeu, J., & Ghahraman, N. (2019). Factors considered by nephrologists in excluding patients from kidney transplant referral. *International Journal of Organ Transplant Medicine, 10*(3). www.ijotm.com

Bolin, J., Bellamy, G., Ferdinand, A., Vuong, A., Kash, B., Schulze, A., & Helduser, J. (2015). Rural healthy people 2020: New decade, same challenges. *The Journal of Rural Health, 31*(3), 326–333. https://doi.org/10.1111/jrh.12116

Borgstrom, D. C., Deveney, K., Hughes, D., Rossi, I. R., Rossi, M. B., Lehman, R., LeMaster, S., & Puls, M. (2022). Rural surgery. *Current Problems in Surgery*, 59(8), 101173. https://doi.org/10.1016/j.cpsurg.2022.101173

Centers for Disease Control and Prevention (CDC). (2017). *Health disparities*. Retrieved September 2, 2023, from www.cdc.gov/aging/disparities/index.htm#:~:text=Health%20 disparities%20are%20preve ntable%20differences,age%20groups%2C%20including%20 older%20adults

Centers for Disease Control and Prevention (CDC). (2022, November 25). *Public health professionals gateway community health assessments & health improvement plans*. Retrieved September 2, 2023, from www.cdc.gov/publichealthgateway/cha/plan.html

Chipp, C., Johnson, M., Brems, C., Warner, T., & Roberts, L. (2008). Adaptations to health care barriers as reported by rural and urban providers. *Journal of Health Care for the Poor and Underserved*, 19(2), 532–549. https://doi.org/10.1353/hpu.0.0002; PMID: 18469424; PMCID: PMC2561996.

Clesse, C., Lighezzolo-Alnot, J., de Lavergne, S., Hamlin, S., & Scheffler, M. (2018). The evolution of birth medicalization: A systematic review. *Midwifery*, 66(67).

Cohen, C., Baird, M., Koirola, N., Kandrack, R., & Martsolf, G. (2021). The surgical and anesthesia workforce and provision of surgical services in rural communities: A mixed-methods examination. *Journal of Rural Health*, 37, 45–54. https://doi.org/10.1111/jrh.12417

Dubay, L., Hill, I., Garrett, B., Blavin, F., Johnston, E., Howell, E., & Cross-Barnet, C. (2020). Improving birth outcomes and lowering costs for women on Medicaid: Impacts of "strong start for mothers and newborns". *Health Affairs*, 39(6), 1042–1050. https://doi.org/10.1377/hlthaff.2019.01042

Gavidia, M. (2021). Underscoring disparities in rural health: Challenges, solutions for a long-standing and growing national issue. *American Journal of Managed Care*. www.ajmc.com/view/underscoring-disparities-in-rural-health-challenges-solutions-for-a-long-standing-and-growing-national-issue

Haldane, V., Chuah, F. L., Srivastava, A., Singh, S. R., Koh, G. C., Seng, C. K., & Legido-Quigley, H. (2019). Community participation in health services development, implementation, and evaluation: A systematic review of empowerment, health, community, and process outcomes. *PLOS One*, 14(5), e0216112. https://doi.org/10.1371/journal.pone.0216112

Health Resources and Services Administration. (2022). *Get started with rural telehealth. Telehealth for rural areas*. Retrieved September 2, 2023, from https://telehealth.hhs.gov/providers/best-practice-guides/telehealth-for-rural-areas/getting-started

Jolles, D., Stapleton, S., Wright, J., Alliman, J., Bauer, K., Townsend, C., & Hoehn-Velasco, L. (2020). Rural resilience: The role of birth centers in the United States. *Birth*, 47(4), 430–437. https://doi.org/10.1111/birt.12516; Epub December 2020 Dec 3. PMID: 33270283; PMCID: PMC7839501.

Lukens, J. (2016). *Freestanding emergency departments: An alternative model for rural communities*. Rural Health Information Hub. Retrieved September 2, 2023, from www.ruralhealthinfo.org/rural-monitor/freestanding-emergency-departments

MacQueen, K., McLellan, E., Metzger, D., Kegeles, S., Strauss, R., Scotti, R., Blanchard, L., & Trotter, R. (2001). What is community? An evidence-based definition for participatory public health. *American Journal of Public Health*, 91(12), 1929–1938. https://doi.org/10.2105/ajph.91.12.1929; PMID: 11726368; PMCID: PMC1446907.

Marmot, M., Bobak, M., & Smith, G. (1995). Explanations for social inequalities in health. In B. C. Amick, S. Levine, A. R. Tarlov, & D. C. Walsh (Eds.), *Society and health* (pp. 172–210). Oxford University Press.

Natafgi, N., Shane, D., Ullrich, F., MacKinney, A., Bell, A., & Ward, M. (2018). Using tele-emergency to avoid patient transfers in rural emergency departments: An assessment of costs and benefits. *Journal of Telemedicine and Telecare*, 24(3), 193–201. https://doi.org/10.1177/1357633X17696585

National Academies of Sciences, Engineering, and Medicine. (2020). *Birth settings in America: Outcomes, quality, access, and choice.* The National Academies Press.

Oki, E., Ota, M., Nakanoko, T., Tanaka, Y., Toyota, S., Hu, Q., Nakaji, Y., Nakanishi, R., Ando, K., Kimura, Y., Hisamatsu, Y., Mimori, K., Takahashi, Y., Morohashi, H., Kanno, T., Tadano, K., Kawashima, K., Takano, H., Ebihara, Y., Shiota, M., Inokuchi, J., Eto, M., Yoshizumi, T., Hakamada, K., Hirano, S., & Mori, M. (2023). Telesurgery and telesurgical support using a double-surgeon cockpit system allowing manipulation from two locations. *Surgical Edoscopy*, 37(8), 6071–6078. https://doi.org/10.1007/s00464-023-10061-6; Epub May 1, 2023. PMID: 37126192; PMCID: PMC10150667.

Olivas, E., Valdez, M., Mufoletto, B, Wallace, J., Stollak, I., & Perry, H. (2023). Reducing inequities in maternal and child health in rural Guatemala through the CBIO+ approach of Curamericas: Management of pregnancy complications at community birthing centers. *International Journal for Equity in Health*, 21(2), 204.

Parker, S., Prince, A., Thomas, L., Song, H., Milosevic, D., & Harris, M. F. (2018). Electronic, mobile, and telehealth tools for vulnerable patients with chronic disease: A systematic review and realist synthesis. *BMJ Open*, 8(8). https://doi.org/10.1136/bmjopen-2017–019192

Sebajang, H., Trudeau, P., Dougall, A., Hegge, S., McKinley, C., & Anvari, M. (2005). Telementoring: An important enabling tool for the community surgeon. *Surgical Innovation*, 12(4), 327–331. https://doi.org/10.1177/155335060501200407. PMID: 16424953.

Shakhnoza, I., & Asalya, A. (2022). Prevention measures of chronic renal failure in adults. *Central Asian Journal of Medical and Natural Science*, 3(4), 87–89. Retrieved September 2, 2023, from https://cajmns.centralasianstudies.org/index.php/CAJMNS/article/view/95

Singh, S., Sharma, V., Patel, P., Anuragi, G., & Sharma, R. G. (2016). Telementoring: An overview and our preliminary experience in the setting up of a cost-effective telementoring facility. *Indian Journal of Surgery*, 78(1), 70–73. https://doi.org/10.1007/s12262-015-1429-y; Epub January 11, 2016. PMID: 27186048; PMCID: PMC4848219.

United States Renal Data System. (2018). *Annual data report.* Retrieved September 28, 2023, from www.usrds.org/annual-data-report/previous-adrs/

5

HEALTHCARE IN THE HOME

Justin Fontenot

Introduction

Considering how to extend patient care services beyond the walls of the hospitals to the home setting continues to increase in popularity and demand in the United States and across the globe. There are many factors driving this phenomenon, the most crucial one being that most people feel overwhelmingly more comfortable receiving healthcare in their homes (Van Leeuwen et al., 2019; Dostálová et al., 2022; Wachterman et al., 2022). Home health care services are also associated with decreased healthcare-related costs (Martin et al., 2021). Increased cost savings and the desire to age-in-place continue to drive the demand for home care services. However, despite its popularity, home care services face many challenges, such as funding, access, and various social determinants, that impact health (Almathami et al., 2020; Brändström et al., 2022).

Furthermore, the United States is currently experiencing challenges related to a growing aging population. Researchers predict that by 2030, people over 65 will account for 20% of the population (Fulmer et al., 2021). Significant advances in the science of medicine and the contemporary

DOI: 10.4324/9781003414902-6

development of advanced pharmaceuticals and cancer-fighting agents have extended the average American lifespan, and people are living longer but with more chronic conditions than ever before (Martin et al., 2021; Johnson, 2021). The rapidly growing aging population poses significant challenges for the healthcare system. As a result of severely limited finite resources which long plagued the American healthcare system, a significant proportion of the aging population will be subjected to disparities in accessing home care services, impacting the mortality of the aging population. This phenomenon calls into question the quality of healthcare services in the United States.

This chapter will cover the various care delivery models for home health care in the United States and the current funding mechanisms for facilitating this growing aspect of healthcare. The chapter will also examine the challenges of delivering services to clients in rural areas and to those with various socioeconomic statuses. The built environment and the impact on health-related outcomes will also be presented. Additionally, there will be an exploration of the various techniques that offer solutions to enhance the inclusivity of home care service delivery in the United States and beyond.

Who Needs Home Care?

In the United States, the needs of those who utilize home care services are diverse, and various health conditions, functional limitations, or age-related needs must be considered. Older adults, people with differing abilities, and those with chronic illnesses require such support. Various levels of care are involved in the delivery of home care services. For example, *home health, hospice, palliative,* and *personal care services* all encompass the broad category of home health care services nationwide.

Home care recipients, particularly older adults, account for a substantial fraction of recipients (Schwartz & Woloshin, 2019). As people age, their physical and cognitive functions may decline, leading to difficulty with performing the *activities of daily living* (ADLs) or *instrumental ADLs* (IADLs) (Chen et al., 2022; Hastaoglu & Mollaoglu, 2022). Home care services can help older individuals maintain independence and morale, enhancing their quality of life. Some of the ways home care models can achieve this are by ensuring assistance with personal care tasks like bathing, cooking, and cleaning; medication management; pain assessment and ongoing management of symptoms; comfort care; spiritual care; social services; and other necessary support (Landers et al., 2016; Askin, 2023).

In addition to older adults, those with differing abilities often receive home care services to meet their specialized health and physical and functional requirements. This population includes people with physical, cognitive, sensory, or intellectual (dis)abilities, necessitating ongoing assistance or intermittent skilled care (Doty et al., 2010; Verlenden et al., 2022). Home care can assist clients with maintaining autonomy and integration into their communities while providing essential medical and personal care (Kaye et al., 2010; Martinsen et al., 2022).

Home care is an essential healthcare service for individuals with chronic illnesses such as heart failure (HF), chronic obstructive pulmonary disease (COPD), or diabetes (Madigan et al., 2012; Li et al., 2022). These patients may require regular monitoring, medication management, or other services to manage their conditions effectively and to avoid exacerbating existing issues or repeat hospitalizations (Russell et al., 2011; Loomer et al., 2022). Home care assistance can also aid these individuals in adhering to client-centered prescribed treatments while maintaining their health and well-being in their homes.

Home Care Service Delivery Options

Various levels of home care services are available for Americans requiring ongoing care. They include home health care, hospice care, personal care services, and palliative care.

Home Health Care

Home health care is a form of specialized care that offers skilled services to homebound clients. Home health services are typically funded under private insurance, Veterans Administration (VA) benefits, Medicare, and Medicaid programs in pay-per-visit or episodic care payment agreements. Under guidelines from the Centers for Medicare and Medicaid Services (CMS), three primary elements warrant approval of funds for home health services to clients (CMS, 2020). Medicaid programs typically follow the same indications for home health services, while private insurance payors vary widely in their reimbursement methods and limitations on visits and other services. These three considerations are very broad, and it is important to note that additional nuance and complexities may change the qualifications for clients receiving home health care services.

First, clients must be under the care of a licensed physician (CMS, 2020). While this may sound fundamental and even reasonably straightforward, many aging clients, especially those in rural areas, lack access to physician care. Despite these challenges, Medicare requires that a licensed physician manage the homebound client's care plan while supervising the services provided by the home care agency. While nurse practitioners (NPs) are prevalent in rural communities supporting primary care, many cannot order home health services or supervise the homebound client's care plan (CMS, 2020).

Second, the client must be homebound (CMS, 2020). This requirement also poses many challenges for home health care providers. Some providers interpret this qualification as meaning that recipients of home health services are not allowed to drive, while others have more lenient interpretations of this regulation. Either way, both pose challenges between providers and regulators and can impact a client's access to care. The idea of homebound status is also highly subjective and nuanced. For example, a client who still drives only to see their physician and to the pharmacy to pick up their medications might also be exhausted after such activity and are primarily confined to their homes.

Lastly, the recipient must require some form of skilled care that is intermittent in duration (CMS, 2020). This requirement is also vague but broad, allowing for a vast range of services provided by skilled clinicians (clinicians licensed in their state to practice their discipline). While skilled care can include wound care, catheter changes, and intravenous infusions, the most critical skilled services are in client education. This means that many home care professionals spend large portions of their day teaching clients not only how to self-manage symptoms related to their chronic illnesses but also the best ways to navigate their homes safely with their specific conditions. Doing so empowers clients to take preventive steps to improve their health and with strategies to remain safe in their homes, thereby reducing hospital stays (Madigan et al., 2012). As one might imagine, skilled services are intentionally broad to meet the specific needs of diverse populations. Clients may qualify for home health care services if they meet all three requirements.

Home health providers must provide the services of skilled clinicians to qualified recipients under the direction and order of the physician. The major skilled disciplines recognized by CMS include the services of registered nurses (RNs), licensed practical nurses (LPNs), physical therapists (PTs), physical therapy assistants (PTAs), occupational therapists (OTs), certified occupational therapy assistants (COTAs), speech therapists (STs), social workers (SWs), and certified nurse assistants (CNAs). The home health client's physician prescribes the duration and frequency of the services. Either way, services must be intermittent and short (30 minutes to 1 hour on average). A typical schedule for a home care client receiving skilled nursing care and physical therapy might involve one weekly visit from the nurse and two to three weekly visits from the PTs. The frequency and duration of services are highly personalized and centered on what is needed to restore the client to independence. Home health care provisioned by CMS and other insurers (Medicaid and private insurance) do not explicitly provide long-term care or extended visiting hours (CMS, 2020). Clients requiring extensive care in the home for extended hours would need another level of care, as these services are not provided (or funded) under the home health care benefit.

There are also various funding mechanisms and models for home health care. The two primary models are either episodic reimbursement or pay-per-visit reimbursement (CMS, 2021). Traditional Medicare patients can receive episodic care based on their individualized needs, while managed Medicare payors, private insurance, and Medicaid provide services by the visit with the duration and frequency depending on the plan's limits and the contracted services with home health care providers. Under the current funding model, disparities exist regarding who receives and accesses home health services.

Hospice Care

Hospice care is often an elusive concept for most people who are trying to understand what it actually entails, with many connecting it with end-of-life care. While this is not an incorrect assumption, there are additional things to consider. The history of hospice in the United States reaches back to the United Kingdom (UK) when Dame Cicely Saunders opened the first hospice (St. Christopher Hospice) in the UK in 1967 (National Hospice and Palliative Care Organization [NHPCO], 2023). The hospice received much support following a famous lecture by Dame Saunders at Yale University in the United States in 1963 (NHPCO, 2023). Close examination of this model in action revealed how specialized care for the terminally ill improved outcomes, providing dignity to recipients of hospice services. Shortly after, Florence Wald and Elisabeth Kubler-Ross advocated for hospice care in 1972, and in 1974, the United States saw the opening of its first hospice in Connecticut (NHPCO, 2023). This hospice, similar to St. Christopher, functioned with volunteer staff and donor funding. In 1982 the U.S. Congress included a provision to fund a hospice benefit for American Medicare beneficiaries, and with this came the first regulations for hospice care, published in the register in 1983 (NHPCO, 2023). Hospice has experienced immense growth since then, and with Medicare-approved funding, the hospice industry saw a massive shift away from nonprofit volunteer-based services to for-profit hospice care services.

Hospice regulations regarding who qualifies for services are straightforward. A client's physician must certify their prognosis as terminal, with end of life expected within six months if the ordinary course of the disease continues untreated (CMS, 2022). While this may sound simplistic, it is actually very broad and complex. Some believe hospice is only reserved for those in the active phase of dying; however, a six-month prognosis does not always indicate immediate death. CMS provides a list of specific chronic diseases that qualify for services with a recommended list of symptoms indicating a functional, emotional, and physical decline. These lists are called *local coverage determinants* (LCDs). These LCDs offer a guide for hospice providers when assessing hospice eligibility. Unlike home care, hospice clients are not required to be homebound. While any disease not listed in the LCDs could result in a terminal prognosis, hospice eligibility also has general requirements providing flexibility for declining clients that do not meet a specific diagnosis covered under the available LCDs. Most hospices report the common hospice diagnoses as congestive heart failure, Alzheimer's disease and other types of dementia, cancers, stroke, and end-stage-kidney disease (NHPCO, 2022). The aging American population continues to drive demand for hospice services. This is evident in the increasing number of beneficiaries receiving hospice care yearly. For example, in 2020, 1.72 million people received hospice care in the United States compared to 1.43 million in 2016 (NHPCO, 2022). Despite this, many Americans continue to die in hospitals.

Many people mistakenly believe that a hospice is an actual structure similar to a hospital. While this was the traditional model of providing hospice care, by and large, the bulk of routine hospice care is delivered in places where clients call home. This could be in long-term care homes, assisted living facilities, private homes, hospital rooms, and in-patient hospice care units, depending on the client's situation. The majority of hospice professionals drive from home to home to care for patients as they near their end of life. Of the major services hospice care providers deliver, the most critical is comfort care through symptom management. Once a client elects the hospice benefit, the hospice provider takes over the care plan for the client related to their primary terminal illness or diagnosis. Under this agreement, the hospice must provide all medications that ease the symptoms associated with the diagnosis, medical equipment (oxygen, mobility items), personal care items, and management of the care plan by the interdisciplinary team, which includes the client and the client's caregivers and/or family members. The frequency and duration of the hospice visit highly depend on the client's needs. The visits may be more frequent as the client declines or experiences a crisis. The medical director (a licensed physician) oversees the care of the hospice census. The registered nurse manages the hospice client's care plan in collaboration with other disciplines, including chaplain/spiritual care services, social services, personal care attendants, and volunteers. Clients can choose which disciplines they need for their care.

Hospice care generally ends with the client's peaceful transition into death. The extent and duration of the service vary and are highly dependent on the client's prognosis, with some clients on service for 12 months and others for a matter of days (if that). Based on the broad and complex matters at the end of life, it might be apparent that disparities continue to occur among dying Americans. Issues like lack of access to services (especially in rural areas), subpar quality of services, limitations in altering homes for hospice care needs, climate change, humid climates prone to disasters like flooding, and funding impact clients across the deep American South and in other rural areas of the country. A summary of the most common methods of funding home care services is provided in Table 5.1.

Personal Care Services

Personal care services is a broad area of elder care in the United States. Personal care usually implies that care is provided by unlicensed (trained and screened) personal care workers. However, these individuals provide critical services to clients living alone, such as bathing, helping with home cleaning, cooking, meal preparation, driving to medical appointments, and companionship. These services are usually delivered in terms of hours, with the number of hours depending on the client's needs. Medicare, some managed Medicare plans, Medicaid, private, and long-term insurance providers fund personal care services. Service-connected veterans and their spouses qualify for funding to assist with personal care or assisted living costs. Overall, the majority of personal care services are paid privately.

There are several models for the delivery of personal care services. Many clients and families prefer to work with agencies that hire and screen

Table 5.1 Summary of the Most Common Funders of Home Care Services

Healthcare Funding	Who Qualifies	How It Is funded	Home Care Services Covered
Medicare	• Age 65 and older • Certain younger individuals with disabilities • People with end-stage renal disease (ESRD)	Funded through payroll taxes, premiums paid by beneficiaries, and general revenue from the federal government	• Part A: Limited home health services (skilled nursing care, physical/occupational/speech therapy) • Part B: Durable medical equipment • Part A and B do not cover personal care services, but Part C (Medicare Advantage) may offer additional benefits
Medicaid	• Individuals and families living with low incomes • Pregnant women • Older adults • People with disabilities	Jointly funded by federal and state governments, with each state administering its own Medicaid program	• Varies by state: May cover home health services (skilled nursing care, therapy), personal care services, and hospice care • Home and community-based services (HCBS) waivers for long-term care
Private insurance	Individuals and families who purchase insurance policies or obtain coverage through their employers	Funded through premiums paid by policyholders and/or their employers	• Coverage varies by plan: May include home health services (skilled nursing care, therapy) and durable medical equipment • Typically does not cover personal care services, but long-term care insurance policies may provide coverage
Managed care	Individuals and families who enroll in health maintenance organizations (HMOs), preferred provider organizations (PPOs), or other types of managed care plans	Funded through premiums paid by policyholders and/or their employers Can also be funded by Medicare part C	• Coverage varies by plan: May include home health services (skilled nursing care, therapy) and durable medical equipment • May offer additional benefits, such as care coordination and case management services • Typically does not cover personal care services, but some plans may provide limited coverage

Adapted from Congressional Research Service. (2022, June). *Who pays for long term services and supports?* Retrieved June 19, 2023, from https://crsreports.congress.gov/product/pdf/IF/IF10343

personal care workers, matching them to clients after thorough consideration of their needs. These agencies usually have workforces that cover geographical areas surrounding the agency. The client or their family makes payment arrangements directly with the personal care agency. While this is a popular framework, many families prefer to work with relatives, community caregivers, and others to provide personal care services to their family members. Under such an arrangement, the client and/or their family will directly pay the caregiver in exchange for their services. This is called private-pay personal care. As with the other home care service options, many people need help to hire private caregivers or personal care agencies due to the cost and limited funding options. While plans like Medicaid offer some limited hours per week, many people require 24-hour care to remain home and out of long-term care facilities.

Palliative Care Services

While hospice care services provide specialized palliative care, they are not the same. Palliative care services are occasionally provided in the same way as other home care services. Some palliative care providers make house calls, but these are limited and depend on the market, making rural areas less likely to deliver these services at home (National Institute on Aging [NIA], 2021). Palliative care services are specialized services where a team specifically trained in palliative treatment options provides symptom management (pain, nausea, spirituality, etc.) for those receiving treatment for serious illnesses. For example, a person with stage I breast cancer receiving chemotherapy treatments with the intention of moving to remission might experience pain, vomiting, nausea, and bowel changes during treatment. Under palliative care services, the team works with the client to relieve the symptoms related to this treatment. A palliative care team typically includes a physician and/or NP, RNs, case managers, and other disciplines to support clients holistically. These services are often found in acute care hospitals, outpatient clients, and some home service providers (NIA, 2021). The main difference between the type of palliative care delivered to hospice patients versus those delivered to nonhospice clients is that palliative care supports the treatment and hopeful remission or reduction of the illness. In contrast, hospice supports the symptoms associated with terminal illness leading to the end of life when no other options exist. See Table 5.2 for a summary of home care services.

Table 5.2 Home Care Delivery Types

Delivery Model	Offered Services	Funding Options	Common Recipients
Hospice care	• Medical care and symptom management for terminally ill patients • Emotional, psychological, and spiritual support • Support and counseling for the patient's family • Bereavement support after death	• Medicare • Medicaid (in most states) • Most private insurance plans • Self-pay or sliding-scale fees depending on the hospice provider	• Patients with a life expectancy of six months or less (as determined by a physician) • Patient and their family must choose comfort care over curative treatments
Home health care	• Skilled nursing care • Physical, occupational, and speech therapy • Medical social services • Home health aide services • Medical equipment and supplies	• Medicare • Medicaid (in some states) • Most private insurance plans • Self-pay	• Patients must be under the care of a physician • Must have a physician's order for home health services • Homebound status or significant difficulty leaving home • Need for intermittent skilled care
Personal care services	• Assistance with activities of daily living (ADLs), such as bathing, dressing, and grooming • Assistance with instrumental activities of daily living (IADLs), such as meal preparation, housekeeping, and medication reminders • Companionship and social interaction	• Medicaid (in some states, under specific waiver programs) • Long-term care insurance • Self-pay • Some local or state-funded programs	• Individuals who need assistance with ADLs and IADLs due to disability, chronic illness, or age-related limitations • No specific medical criteria required

(Continued)

Table 5.2 (Continued)

Delivery Model	Offered Services	Funding Options	Common Recipients
Palliative care services	• Symptom and pain management for patients with serious illnesses • Emotional and psychological support for patients and their families • Assistance with care coordination and communication among healthcare providers • Support in navigating medical decision-making	• Medicare (for specific services) • Medicaid (in some states) • Most private insurance plans • Self-pay	• Patients with serious, chronic, or life-threatening illnesses • Can be provided at any stage of illness and alongside curative treatments

(National Association for Home Care and Hospice. (2023, December). *Home care and hospice basics.* Retrieved June 19, 2023, from www.nahc.org/consumers-information/home-care-hospice-basics/

Now that the reader has a working knowledge of the various types of home care delivery models, the people who need this care, the services offered, and the accessibility challenges, let us look at a few case studies, followed by some discussion questions.

CASE STUDY 1

A discharge planner is caring for a 72-year-old male client recovering from an acute heart failure exacerbation. He received intense fluid management monitoring during his hospital stay and was given diuretics to improve his breathing. Over the hospital stay, the staff became concerned with how weak the client had become. The physician ordered physical therapy, and now the client is doing better, but he still experiences some weakness and is confused about his medications. The client lives alone in a single-story (but small) home in a small rural community and had minimal issues before this hospital stay. His daughter lives approximately three hours away but visits often.

DISCUSSION QUESTIONS

- What type of services do you think this client qualifies for?
- What barriers to care delivery do you foresee for this client?

CASE STUDY 2

You are visiting with an older neighbor, and during your visit, you note your neighbor's struggle to walk. Your neighbor appears disheveled in their appearance. This is a new development, as you often visit your neighbor. When you offer concern, your neighbor tells you that their back pain has become unbearable and they cannot help themselves with bathing and laundry. They also inform you that they are living on a limited income and, due to the current state of inflation, are having trouble paying for basic medical needs like visits to the physician and pain medication.

DISCUSSION QUESTIONS

- What services might you recommend for your neighbor?
- What are some of the barriers to accessing the care you suggested?

Significant Challenges to Home Care Delivery

Geographic and Transportation Challenges

Several aspects of the client's built environment pose challenges for home care delivery. The first involves geographic location and transportation challenges. Rural areas especially lack home care providers, and formal transportation systems limit service access (Bazargan & Bazargan-Hejazi, 2021). A lack of sufficient *infrastructure* (poor roadways, bridges, and a lack of pavement) coupled with poor socioeconomic status makes transportation to medical appointments and healthcare professionals travel time increase costs and limit services to such areas. Marginalized communities experience the most disparities, often resulting from *structural and systemic issues* (Bazargan & Bazargan-Hejazi, 2021). Geographical challenges frequently impact rural communities. Often lacking the funding (taxes, business income, well-equipped school systems, and community support) to build better roadways, provide accessible public transportation, and expand basic technology to operate businesses, rural communities face ongoing challenges with access to healthcare services.

Housing Conditions and Accessibility

Another significant barrier involves housing conditions and accessibility. People who live in poverty, such as those who live in the American South, often live in homes in various states of disrepair (Patel et al., 2020). Older homes often need more attention, with ongoing repairs and maintenance presenting many challenges for healthcare delivery in the home. These repairs can range in cost, and people living on fixed incomes (older people and people with disabilities) may not have the money necessary to keep up with repairs. Some of the challenges related to care delivery involve such issues as leaky roofs, soft flooring (for homes that are elevated, common in coastal subtropical humid climates), limited space for medical equipment, general lack of modern technology (computers, internet, cable access), and heating/cooling challenges (Bedney et al., 2010; Grant et al., 2022).

These challenges not only pose safety hazards for clients but can also impact the safety of the professionals delivering the care. States with sub-standard infrastructure, such as the lack of paved roads or roads and bridges in disrepair, can limit the ability of home care professionals to reach the client promptly. In coastal communities, it is not uncommon to encounter situations where a boat might be required to reach the client's home. These situations can limit the access of professionals and the safe delivery of *durable medical equipment* (DME) to the client's home – a significant barrier to the delivery of the necessary supplies for the patient/client. Homes with outdated electrical systems can pose safety hazards for clients and visiting staff. Supporting cost-saving and effective healthcare delivery in the home could be difficult if it requires significant improvements at the structural and accessibility levels.

Socioeconomic Factors

Communities that lack access to resources often live below the poverty line, have underfunded public education institutions, and have high unemployment rates (Cyr et al., 2019). Additionally, low-income communities have substandard health outcomes compared to people with more financial resources and access to care (Cyr et al., 2019). In the United States, many communities rely on home care providers with locally owned practices that require funding, resources, and committees with qualified personnel to provide adequate services to clients. Socioeconomic factors are wide-reaching and significantly impact not just the accessibility of care but also the essential foundations needed to operate businesses that care for clients.

Ongoing systemic barriers such as racism and discrimination impact access to housing and resources, continuing to marginalized communities, many of which are communities of color (McMaughan et al., 2020). The socioeconomic status of the community impacts the ability to build better roads, neighborhoods, affordable housing, healthcare centers, home care agencies, and educational centers, all of which lead to suboptimal healthcare outcomes that impact communities broadly. Addressing issues that impact the socioeconomic status of communities involves legislative and policy changes to improve access, resources, and, eventually, the health and well-being of communities living in unfavorable socioeconomic conditions.

Climate Change

Climate change is a growing challenge globally, especially among those residing in coastal subtropical areas (Ebi et al., 2021). Increased weather events and climate disasters continue to impact communities, destroying infrastructure and critical public health and community-based healthcare services. Older homes and homes exposed to high humidity levels, common in the South and coastal communities, require ongoing repair and maintenance. Homes built before the era of climate change – the *Anthropocene* – are not adequately constructed to withstand hurricane-force wind, excessive flooding, roof issues, tornados, and heavy rainfall and have poorly insulated walls, windows, and door jams. Critical staff shortages impacting wait times and emergent care tend to occur because healthcare workers residing in these communities are also impacted by weather events and disasters (Ebi et al., 2021).

Rising sea levels, poor drainage systems, and outdated pump equipment can destroy buildings, communities, infrastructure, community resources, and healthcare systems. The inability to access clients in their homes during emergencies, power outages, and other weather-related crises leave many communities undersourced. Consequently, health outcomes are negatively impacted, and disparities among socioeconomically disadvantaged communities increase. Ongoing support and high-level legislation are urgently needed to mitigate the impacts of climate crises. Now we will look at another case study and review discussion questions.

CASE STUDY 3

A client in rural coastal south Louisiana recently experienced flooding from drenching Gulf-induced rainfall. Once the client realized how rapidly the water was rising without any foreseeable break in the rain, they contacted emergency services. Unfortunately, emergency services could not access the home during the flooding event. The client used an axe to make a hole in the roof and waited for emergency services to rescue them. The client has a history of chronic obstructive pulmonary disease (COPD) from working in the salt mines. Since the electricity went out during the event, the client went for an extended period without oxygen. The client also suffered sunburn to their upper extremities. The client spent a few days in the hospital and was transferred to a shelter.

DISCUSSION QUESTIONS

- What home care services should this client receive following this traumatic event?
- What climate factors influenced the client's ability to care for themselves in their home?
- What can communities do to rebuild their homes and continue with medical treatments despite emergencies like these?

Recommended Solutions

While many solutions are available, addressing significant challenges to home care delivery will require large-scale efforts. Table 5.3 summarizes suggested solutions for meeting ongoing challenges and delivering critical home care services to those who need them most.

Table 5.3 Summary of Recommended Solutions for Major Challenges Impacting Home Care

Challenges	Possible Solutions
Geographic and transportation issues	• Expand telehealth services to reach remote areas. • Offer mobile health clinics for in-home care. • Provide transportation assistance for patients and caregivers. • Partner with local community organizations to increase care accessibility.
Housing and accessibility	• Implement home modification programs to improve accessibility. • Offer financial assistance for home repairs and upgrades. • Develop affordable, accessible housing options for seniors and individuals with disabilities. • Educate caregivers and patients about available resources and services.
Socioeconomic challenges	• Increase funding and resources for home care services in underserved communities. • Offer sliding-scale fees or financial assistance programs for low-income patients.

(Continued)

Table 5.3 (Continued)

Challenges	Possible Solutions
	• Improve access to healthcare through outreach and education initiatives. • Strengthen community-based organizations to support home care service delivery.
Climate change	• Develop emergency preparedness plans for home care providers and patients. • Offer education and training for caregivers on climate change–related health risks. • Implement energy-efficient measures in homes to reduce utility costs and environmental impact. • Advocate for policies addressing climate change and its impact on healthcare delivery.

Adapted from:

Bazargan, M., & Bazargan-Hejazi, S. (2021). Disparities in palliative and hospice care and completion of advance care planning and directives among non-Hispanic blacks: A scoping review of recent literature. *American Journal of Hospice and Palliative Medicine, 38*(6), 688–718. https://doi.org/10.1177/1049909120966585;

Bedney, B. J., Goldberg, R. B., & Josephson, K. (2010). Aging in place in naturally occurring retirement communities: Transforming aging through supportive service programs. *Journal of Housing for the Elderly, 24*(3–4), 304–321. https://doi.org/10.1080/02763893.2010.522455;

Cyr, M. E., Etchin, A. G., Guthrie, B. J., & Benneyan, J. C. (2019). Access to specialty healthcare in urban versus rural US populations: A systematic literature review. *BMC Health Services Research, 19*(1), 974. https://doi.org/10.1186/s12913-019-4815-5;

Ebi, K. L., Vanos, J., Baldwin, J. W., Bell, J. E., Hondula, D. M., Errett, N. A., Hayes, K., Reid, C. E., Saha, S., Spector, J., & Berry, P. (2021). Extreme weather and climate change: Population health and health system implications. *Annual Review of Public Health, 42*(1), 293–315. https://doi.org/10.1146/annurev-publhealth-012420-105026.

Definitions

ADLs (activities of daily living): Essential tasks for basic self-care, such as bathing, dressing, eating, toileting, and mobility.

The **Anthropocene,** suggested as a new geological epoch, denotes the significant impact of human activities on Earth's ecosystems and climate.

In **client-centered care**, healthcare providers prioritize meeting individuals' unique needs, preferences, and values while emphasizing communication and collaboration between patients and doctors.

Home health care services involve medical and nonmedical assistance provided directly within clients' homes, such as skilled nursing care, therapy sessions, and support for daily living activities.

Hospice: A type of specialized care for those facing terminal illness, designed to offer comfort and support to patients and their families instead of curative treatments.

Instrumental activities of daily living (IADLs): Daily tasks requiring more sophisticated skills, including meal preparation, housecleaning, shopping for essential items such as medication management, and transportation.

Infrastructure refers to any physical support network necessary for operation within an organization or community; examples include roads, buildings, and utilities that ensure smooth running.

Medicaid: Administered jointly by federal and state health authorities, offers health coverage to low-income individuals and families as well as pregnant women, older adults, and people living with disabilities.

Medicare: A federal health insurance program that offers coverage to people 65 or over, younger individuals living with disabilities, and those diagnosed with end-stage renal disease.

Palliative care: Specialized medical assistance designed to alleviate symptoms and enhance the quality of life for people suffering from severe, chronic, or life-threatening illnesses.

Personal care services: Nonmedical assistance with activities of daily living (ADLs) and instrumental ADLs for individuals living with disabilities, chronic illnesses, or age-related functional or physical limitations.

Private health insurance: Coverage provided through private companies, either individually or employer-sponsored plans.

Systemic issues/barriers: Deeply embedded problems within systems that impact many individuals or groups and require structural modifications to solve.

VA benefits: Veterans Affairs (VA) provides healthcare services, disability compensation payments, and education assistance for eligible veterans and their families through its department.

References

Almathami, H. K. Y., Win, K. T., & Vlahu-Gjorgievska, E. (2020). Barriers and facilitators that influence telemedicine-based, real-time, online consultation at patients' homes: Systematic literature review. *Journal of Medical Internet Research, 22*(2), e16407. https://doi. org/10.2196/16407

Askin, E. (2023). *Health care handbook a clear and concise guide to the United States health care system.* Wolters Kluwer Medical.

Bazargan, M., & Bazargan-Hejazi, S. (2021). Disparities in palliative and hospice care and completion of advance care planning and directives among non-hispanic blacks: A scoping review of recent literature. *American Journal of Hospice and Palliative Medicine, 38*(6), 688–718. https://doi.org/10.1177/1049909120966585

Bedney, B. J., Goldberg, R. B., & Josephson, K. (2010). Aging in place in naturally occurring retirement communities: Transforming aging through supportive service programs. *Journal of Housing for the Elderly, 24*(3–4), 304–321. https://doi.org/10.1080/02 763893.2010.522455

Brändström, A., Meyer, A. C., Modig, K., & Sandström, G. (2022). Determinants of home care utilization among the Swedish old: Nationwide register-based study. *European Journal of Ageing, 19*(3), 651–662. https://doi.org/10.1007/s10433-021-00669-9

Centers for Medicare and Medicaid Services. (2020). *Medicare benefit policy manual chapter 7-home health services.* Retrieved June 19, 2023, from www.cms.gov/Regulations-and-Guidance/Guidance/Manuals/downloads/bp102c07.pdf

Centers for Medicare and Medicaid Services. (2021). *Home health prospective payment system (HH PPS).* Retrieved June 19, 2023, from www.cms.gov/Medicare/Medicare-Fee-for-Service-Payment/HomeHealthPPS

Centers for Medicare and Medicaid Services. (2022). *Hospice.* Retrieved June 19, 2023, from www.cms.gov/Medicare/Medicare-Fee-for-Service-Payment/Hospice

Chen, S., Jones, L. A., Jiang, S., Jin, H., Dong, D., Chen, X., Wang, D., Zhang, Y., Xiang, L., Zhu, A., & Cardinal, R. N. (2022). Difficulty and help with activities of daily living among older adults living alone during the COVID-19 pandemic: A multi-country population-based study. *BMC Geriatrics, 22*(1), 181. https://doi.org/10.1186/s12877-022-02799-w

Congressional Research Service. (2022, June). *Who pays for long term services and supports?* Retrieved June 19, 2023, from https://crsreports.congress.gov/product/pdf/IF/IF10343

Cyr, M. E., Etchin, A. G., Guthrie, B. J., & Benneyan, J. C. (2019). Access to specialty healthcare in urban versus rural US populations: A systematic literature review. *BMC Health Services Research, 19*(1), 974. https://doi.org/10.1186/s12913-019-4815-5

Dostálová, V., Bártová, A., Bláhová, H., & Holmerová, I. (2022). The experiences and needs of frail older people receiving home health care: A qualitative study. *International Journal of Older People Nursing, 17*(1). https://doi.org/10.1111/opn.12418

Doty, P., Mahoney, K. J., & Sciegaj, M. (2010). New state strategies to meet long-term care needs. *Health Affairs, 29*(1), 49–56. https://doi.org/10.1377/hlthaff.2009.0521

Ebi, K. L., Vanos, J., Baldwin, J. W., Bell, J. E., Hondula, D. M., Errett, N. A., Hayes, K., Reid, C. E., Saha, S., Spector, J., & Berry, P. (2021). Extreme weather and climate change: Population health and health system implications. *Annual Review of Public Health, 42*(1), 293–315. https://doi.org/10.1146/annurev-publhealth-012420-105026

Fulmer, T., Reuben, D. B., Auerbach, J., Fick, D. M., Galambos, C., & Johnson, K. S. (2021). Actualizing better health and health care for older adults: Commentary describes six vital directions to improve the care and quality of life for all older Americans. *Health Affairs*, 40(2), 219–225. https://doi.org/10.1377/hlthaff.2020.01470

Grant, T., Croce, E., & Matsui, E. C. (2022). Asthma and the social determinants of health. *Annals of Allergy, Asthma & Immunology*, 128(1), 5–11. https://doi.org/10.1016/j.anai.2021.10.002

Hastaoglu, F., & Mollaoglu, M. (2022). The effects of activities of daily living education on the independence and life satisfaction of elders. *Perspectives in Psychiatric Care*, 58(4), 2978–2985. https://doi.org/10.1111/ppc.13149

Johnson, S. (2021). *Extra life: A short history of living longer*. Riverhead Books.

Kaye, H. S., Harrington, C., & LaPlante, M. P. (2010). Long-term care: Who gets it, who provides it, who pays, and how much? *Health Affairs*, 29(1), 11–21. https://doi.org/10.1377/hlthaff.2009.0535

Landers, S., Madigan, E., Leff, B., Rosati, R. J., McCann, B. A., Hornbake, R., MacMillan, R., Jones, K., Bowles, K., Dowding, D., Lee, T., Moorhead, T., Rodriguez, S., & Breese, E. (2016). The future of home health care: A strategic framework for optimizing value. *Home Health Care Management & Practice*, 28(4), 262–278. https://doi.org/10.1177/1084822316666368

Li, Y., Fang, J., Li, M., & Luo, B. (2022). Effect of nurse-led hospital-to-home transitional care interventions on mortality and psychosocial outcomes in adults with heart failure: A meta-analysis. *European Journal of Cardiovascular Nursing*, 21(4), 307–317. https://doi.org/10.1093/eurjcn/zvab105

Loomer, L., Rahman, M., Mroz, T. M., Gozalo, P. L., & Mor, V. (2022). Impact of higher payments for rural home health episodes on rehospitalizations. *The Journal of Rural Health*, 39(3). https://doi.org/10.1111/jrh.12725

Madigan, E. A., Gordon, N. H., Fortinsky, R. H., Koroukian, S. M., Piña, I., & Riggs, J. S. (2012). Rehospitalization in a national population of home health care patients with heart failure. *Health Services Research*, 47(6), 2316–2338. https://doi.org/10.1111/j.1475-6773.2012.01416.x

Martin, A. B., Hartman, M., Lassman, D., Catlin, A., & The National Health Expenditure Accounts Team. (2021). National health care spending in 2019: Steady growth for the fourth consecutive year: Study examines national health care spending for 2019. *Health Affairs*, 40(1), 14–24. https://doi.org/10.1377/hlthaff.2020.02022

Martinsen, B., Norlyk, A., & Gramstad, A. (2022). The experience of dependence on homecare among people ageing at home. *Ageing and Society*, 1–16. https://doi.org/10.1017/S0144686X22000150

McMaughan, D. J., Oloruntoba, O., & Smith, M. L. (2020). Socioeconomic status and access to healthcare: Interrelated drivers for healthy aging. *Frontiers in Public Health*, 8, 231. https://doi.org/10.3389/fpubh.2020.00231

National Association for Home Care and Hospice. (2023, December). *Home care and hospice basics*. Retrieved June 19, 2023, from www.nahc.org/consumers-information/home-care-hospice-basics/

National Hospice and Palliative Care Organization. (2022). *Hospice facts and figures*. Retrieved June 19, 2023, from www.nhpco.org/hospice-care-overview/hospice-facts-figures/

National Hospice and Palliative Care Organization. (2023). *History of hospice*. Retrieved June 19, 2023, from www.nhpco.org/hospice-care-overview/history-of-hospice/

National Institute on Aging. (2021). *What are palliative and hospice care?* Retrieved June 19, 2023, from www.nia.nih.gov/health/what-are-palliative-care-and-hospice-care#:~:text=setting%20 for%20care.-,What%20is%20palliative%20care%3F,to%20cure%20their%20serious%20 illness

Patel, J. A., Nielsen, F. B. H., Badiani, A. A., Assi, S., Unadkat, V. A., Patel, B., Ravindrane, R., & Wardle, H. (2020). Poverty, inequality and COVID-19: The forgotten vulnerable. *Public Health*, 183, 110–111. https://doi.org/10.1016/j.puhe.2020.05.006

Russell, D., Rosati, R. J., Sobolewski, S., Marren, J., & Rosenfeld, P. (2011). Implementing a transitional care program for high-risk heart failure patients: Findings from a community-based partnership between a certified home healthcare agency and regional hospital. *Journal for Healthcare Quality*, 33(6), 17–24. https://doi.org/10.1111/ j.1945-1474.2011.00167.x

Schwartz, L. M., & Woloshin, S. (2019). Medical marketing in the United States, 1997– 2016. *JAMA*, 321(1), 80. https://doi.org/10.1001/jama.2018.19320

Van Leeuwen, K. M., Van Loon, M. S., Van Nes, F. A., Bosmans, J. E., De Vet, H. C. W., Ket, J. C. F., Widdershoven, G. A. M., & Ostelo, R. W. J. G. (2019). What does quality of life mean to older adults? A thematic synthesis. *PLOS One*, 14(3), e0213263. https:// doi.org/10.1371/journal.pone.0213263

Verlenden, J. V., Zablotsky, B., Yeargin-Allsopp, M., & Peacock, G. (2022). Healthcare access and utilization for young adults with disability: U. S., 2014–2018. *Journal of Adolescent Health*, 70(2), 241–248. https://doi.org/10.1016/j.jadohealth.2021.08.023

Wachterman, M. W., Luth, E. A., Semco, R. S., & Weissman, J. S. (2022). Where Americans die – Is there really "no place like home"? *New England Journal of Medicine*, 386(11), 1008–1010. https://doi.org/10.1056/NEJMp2112297

Part 2

GENERAL PRINCIPLES FOR THE DESIGN OF EQUITABLE, INCLUSIVE HEALTHCARE SETTINGS AND INNOVATIONS IN THE DESIGN OF HEALTHCARE SPACES

6

CONSIDERATIONS FOR THE DESIGN OF HEALTHCARE FACILITIES ACROSS MULTIPLE SCALES

PART I: HEALTHCARE ENVIRONMENTAL CONTROL SYSTEMS AND SAFETY

Denise M. Linton and Kiwana T. McClung

Introduction

Environmental control systems are an important consideration for design and planning teams seeking to implement inclusive healthcare facilities. Healthcare facilities house essential services, and interruptions to the systems needed to meet healthcare needs could be devastating for communities. System interruptions are not the only critical consideration for healthcare facilities; how these systems perform is also of concern. Systems that do not work properly could facilitate the spread of infectious airborne illness or worsen existing illnesses. There have even been recorded instances of buildings that make people sick, a condition attributed to improperly installed or maintained heating, ventilation, and air conditioning (HVAC) systems. Thus,

DOI: 10.4324/9781003414902-8

environmental control systems are an important consideration for designers, planners, and healthcare administrators during the design, construction, and renovation process. The considerations in this chapter will reference these systems, their role in cultivating inclusive healthcare environments, and important considerations for their integration into healthcare facilities.

Heating, Ventilation, and Air Conditioning Systems

Healthcare facilities administrators need to ensure that patients are cared for in a safe environment that minimizes the spread of disease and sickness. These environments should also be designed so that they facilitate an ideal environment for healthcare professionals to care for patients with a variety of issues. Beyond the spatial, these environments must consider temperature, light, air, and sound – elements that promote healing in spaces while preventing the growth of the harmful. Such is the case with HVAC systems in healthcare facilities. Not only are these systems designed to create thermal comfort or protection from the exterior, they are also designed to control airflow, mitigate the spread of infection, and minimize the growth of harmful bacteria. Considerations for negative and positive pressure rooms to control infection will be discussed next.

Negative and Positive Pressure Rooms

Healthcare facilities can maintain a safe environment in a variety of ways. The primary goal is to avert the spread of pollutants that cause infection by maintaining a sterile space/room or limiting access using negative and positive pressure rooms (Air Innovations, 2023). In negative pressure rooms, the air pressure inside the room is lowered so that the air outside can enter the room and the air in the room cannot leave via the HVAC system. Consequently, infectious agents/pollutants are kept within the room and persons outside are not exposed (Braude & Femling, 2020). While airborne isolation may be the intention with negative pressure rooms, there are other areas where negative pressure could be a benefit, preventing the spread of contaminants. These spaces include waiting rooms, areas where triaging occurs, bathrooms, and areas for laundry that is soiled. In addition to preventing potentially contaminated air from escaping, these rooms are equipped with either exhaust systems that direct the air in the space to the exterior or highly efficient particulate air filters. Although these systems are effective in containing air within a space, healthcare professionals caring for patients within these spaces should still wear personal protective equipment, as the recommended number of air exchanges per hour for these airborne isolation spaces is 12 per hour. Consequently, upwards of 35 minutes is required for air removal efficiency at 99% (Braude & Femling, 2020).

On the other hand, in positive pressure rooms, the pressure in the environment is lower than that in the room. Therefore, the air that escapes from the room does not return, getting rid of infectious agents/pollutants; patients who are at high risk for disease and infection are protected (Air Innovations, 2023). This is particularly important in the nursery (animal and human), operating theater, and laboratories for in vitro fertilization. It is important for administration to collaborate with planners since such rooms require:

• High-efficiency particulate absorbing (HEPA) filters through which air should recirculate, thereby controlling pollutants that are in the air.
• An entryway that self-closes and has a seal.
• Windows, walls, ceilings, and floors that are completely sealed.
• Movement of air in the directions that one wishes by using, for example, a fan and ductwork.
• A system that monitors the pressure so that it can be adjusted.
• A space between the room and its surroundings to facilitate the delivery of items, observation by staff, and to store protective equipment.
• Ultraviolet radiation can also be used to maintain an environment that is sterile. For example this system reduces viruses, such as coronavirus, in the room and protects the staff who enters the room (Air Innovations, 2023).

Finally, planning teams need to ensure that the rooms that are pressurized align with the space and needs of the setting, that the legal regulations are adhered to, and that the room completely protects everyone from diseases that are infectious (Braude & Femling, 2020).

Heating, Ventilation, and Air Conditioning System

There are many best practices and considerations for the HVAC system in a new design and one that is undergoing major renovations. The spread of airborne diseases, such as tuberculosis, can be controlled or slowed by the

HVAC system. Therefore, the design team needs to adhere to regulations; federal laws; local municipalities; executive orders; and the needs of all end users, architects/engineers, and other team members (International Health Facility Guidelines [IHFG], 2020). Some specific considerations include:

- Provide the expected comfort and function.
- The safety of patients and infection control – for example, ensure that air does not recirculate and mechanical filtration is in accordance with the correct rating. Separate air handling units to prevent cross contamination, for example, main kitchen, operating theater, and the mortuary.
- Comply with the code requirement for hourly changes to the air.
- Modifiable and expandable.
- Determine all regulations, standards, and guidelines and adhere to them, especially local standards.
- Location – major equipment should be preferably in a mechanical room; however, exhaust and smoke management fans can be located outside the facility. In temperate or cold regions, major equipment should not be located on the roof or exposed to the air.
- Fire safety is part of this consideration (IHFG, 2020).
- Maintenance.
- Specific requirements for each space, including, laboratories, pharmacy, rooms where imaging (ultrasound, radiologic studies, magnetic resonance imaging [MRI]) occurs, patient rooms, critical care rooms in intensive care units, and isolation rooms. (Note: The design of HVACs in the outpatient setting is different from the inpatient/hospital setting.)

Effects of HVAC Failure

Since the HVAC in hospitals filters, cools, humidifies, dehumidifies, and manages the pressure regimen, failure can result in no pressure in rooms and spaces and subsequent risk to patients who are immune-compromised and viral infection spread. These systems should be *reliable, redundant, and resilient* (IHFG, 2020, pp. 16–17). *Reliability* refers to the functioning of all parts of the system, including its installation and maintenance. Those who are purchasing the system should be actively involved with the manufacturer in all aspects, beginning with the design. *Redundancy* refers to the system that will be used if or when the main system fails. *Resiliency* refers to whether and how the system will continue to function if some of its parts fail. Healthcare facilities such as hospitals need to be proactive against hail, sand, or snow storms in addition to heavy rain, which are becoming quite common. Consider the sound of the HVAC system and any generator that is used during an outage and place it in an area where people will not be negatively impacted.

Safe Water

The water that is available to clients and patrons in all healthcare facilities needs to be free of contaminants that can result in illnesses depicted in Table 6.1. The potential problems can be averted by testing and treating water according to standards and guidelines, corrosion and leak prevention, and replacing lead pipes, if present.

Table 6.1 Water Contaminants and Their Effects

Contaminants	Effects
High lead levels	Children – low growth and intelligent quotient, impaired hearing, disease of the cardiovascular system, and problems with behavior Adults – hypertension, disease of the kidney and heart, and problems with fertility
Per- and polyfluoroalkyl (PFAS)	Cancer of the testicles and kidney, reduced vaccine effectiveness, developmental abnormalities of fetuses, liver and thyroid disorders
Atrazine	Pesticide – especially a problem in water of the Midwest and Southern United States and causes disruption of the endocrine system
Pathogens	Parasites, bacteria (*Escherichia coli* leading to Legionnaires' disease), and viruses
By-products of chlorine treatment, for example, trihalomethanes	Cancer and disorders of the reproductive system at elevated levels

Source: (MacMillan, 2023).

Hazardous Waste Disposal

Healthcare administrators, planners, and designers need to consider the management of their waste because historically, adequate staff training does not occur, systems need to be in place, and sufficient funds and resources are not allocated, and neither are regulations adhered to (World Health Organization [WHO], 2018). Hazardous waste can also contaminate water if it is not treated before disposal and/or placed in improperly constructed landfills.

Globally, approximately 15% of the waste that is produced by healthcare facilities is considered to be hazardous materials that are harmful to their patients, staff, and the public (WHO, 2018). This waste primarily originates from healthcare facilities such as hospitals, nursing homes, laboratories, autopsies, mortuaries, and research centers, in addition to blood banks. Harmful waste that healthcare facilities generate include infectious, pathologic, sharps, chemical, pharmaceutical, cytotoxic, and radioactive waste. Although a problem for everyone, people in low-income countries rarely separate their "hazardous waste" and are at high risk for the deleterious effects of these hazardous materials. Some effects are burns from chemicals used to sterilize and disinfect and injuries related to sharps, for example, hepatitis B, hepatitis C, and HIV. Worldwide, approximately 16 billion injections are given annually; however, only some of the used syringes and needles are discarded correctly. Unfortunately, these waste materials are usually burnt in an incinerator or open fire and they sometimes emit harmful substances, such as "dioxins and furans" (WHO, 2018). To reduce and prevent the harmful effects of hazardous waste, health facilities should:

- Develop strategies to reduce the amount of waste that is produced and separate hazardous waste from nonhazardous waste
- Gradually build a system that is comprehensive and addresses responsibilities, the allocation of resources, and how to handle and dispose of waste based on both international and national requirements
- Educate about the potential harmful effects of hazardous waste
- Implement safety measures to collect, handle, store, transport, treat, and dispose of waste
- When possible, autoclave, microwave, or treat chemically instead of incinerating medical waste (WHO, 2018)

Power

Loss of electricity is a worldwide problem that is increasing in frequency because of natural disasters that are a result of climate change, in addition to electricity grids that have been in place for a long time (Casey et al., 2020). The negative health consequences of these outages include poisoning from carbon monoxide; illnesses related to temperature; and hospitalization for heart, lung, and kidney disease, particularly in people whose medical equipment requires electricity. According to Casey et al., the two groups that are at the highest risks are children and the elderly.

"System failures in February 2021 left 100,000 residents without water for weeks during the same winter storm that crippled the Texas grid. Storms brought 4 inches of snow, 2 inches of sleet, and multiple days of subfreezing temperatures to Mississippi, causing power outages and equipment failure at Jackson's water-treatment plant. Mechanisms that could have prevented system failures during a winter storm weren't in place" (Mizelle, 2023, p. 2213).

Communications Systems

Communication technologies, which ease the ability to disseminate information to those who need it most, is a critical consideration in the design of inclusive healthcare spaces. Poor communications in healthcare settings could not only create inequities in the care of patients but could also compromise the safety of healthcare professionals. Interestingly, Coiera (2006) suggests that if the concept of communicative information exchange is conceived of as a space, based upon the total number of informational and interpersonal transactions, one could determine the efficiency of a facility's communication space. The size of a facility or number of individuals working within that facility does not matter if there is an adequate communication system in place.

The establishment of "communication channels" is essential and can take on several forms. Telecommunications like email and the telephone serve as common communication channels in healthcare settings, allowing for two-way synchronous communication. Automated telephone communication systems (ATCSs) take this concept a step further, allowing for the exchange of healthcare information between patients and healthcare professionals. ATCSs also have the ability to exchange voicemail messages between patients and providers through their own devices (Posadzki et al., 2016). There are also asynchronous methods of communication, like message boards or post-its, but with the rise in technological advances, these methods are becoming less common (Coiera, 2006).

A number of communication services and devices can serve as a part of communication networks. Answering services with formal recorded messages are useful in healthcare settings, as are personal communication devices like smart watches.

Conclusion

Community residents enter healthcare facilities to attain optimal health, but poor environmental control systems can prevent this from occurring. It is important that healthcare facilities at all scales invest in their environmental control systems because the ill effects can be far reaching, from the patients and staff to the people in the communities that they occupy. Furthermore, this issue requires attention because of the unpredictable weather patterns and infectious disease outbreaks that are being experienced worldwide. Fortunately for us, technological advances can be incorporated in the design and planning of new healthcare facilities and those that are being renovated.

References

Air Innovations. (2023). *Negative and positive pressure rooms 101/hospital infection control.* Retrieved October 5, 2023, from https://airinnovations.com/blog/negative-positive-pressure-rooms-hospital-infection-control/

Braude, D., & Femling, J. (2020). Dangerous misperceptions about negative-pressure rooms. *Annals of Emergency Medicine, 76*(5), 690. https//doi.org/10.1016/j.annemergmed.2020.05.036

Casey, J. A., Fukurai, M., Hernandez, D., Balsari, S., & Kiang, M. V. (2020). Power outages and community health: A narrative review. *Current Environmental Health Report, 7*(4), 371–383. https//doi.org/10.1007/s40572-020-00295-0

Coiera, E. (2006). Communication systems in healthcare. *Clinical Biochemist Reviews, 27*(2), 89–98.

International Health Facility Guidelines. (2020). *Mechanical (HVAC) engineering design.* Retrieved October 5, 2023, from www.healthfacilityguidelines.com/ViewPDF/ViewIndexPDF/Mechanical_HVAC_Engineering_Design

MacMillan, A. (2023). *Safe drinking water: What's in your drinking water?* Retrieved October 4, 2023, from www.nrdc.org/stories/whats-your-drinking-water

Mizelle, R. M. (2023). A slow-moving disaster – The Jackson water crisis and the health effects of racism. *New England Journal of Medicine*, 388(24), 2212–2214. https://doi.org/10.1056/NEJMp2212978

Posadzki, P., Mastellos, N., Ryan, R., Gunn, L. H., Felix, L. M., Pappas, Y., Gagnon, M. P., Julious, S., Xiang, L., Oldenburg, B., & Car, J. (2016). Automated telephone communication systems for preventative healthcare and management of long-term conditions. *Cochrane Database Systematic Review*, 12. https//doi.org/10.1002/14651858.CD009921.pub2

World Health Organization (WHO). (2018, February 8). *Health-care waste*. Retrieved October 12, 2023, from www.who.int/news-room/fact-sheets/detail/health-care-waste

7

CONSIDERATIONS FOR THE DESIGN OF HEALTHCARE FACILITIES ACROSS MULTIPLE SCALES

PART II: THE HEALTHCARE EXPERIENCE

Kristi L. Anderson

There are many ways in which individuals describe and use healthcare facilities. To say that healthcare facilities are primarily a place for the unwell, however, only acknowledges a certain aspect of the healthcare experience. Indeed, they can be described as places where individuals and families seek care and treatment for acute and chronic illnesses. They ensure that individuals and their families receive services for health promotion and the prevention of illnesses. Healthcare facilities can also support spirituality and transcendence for those that are in their journey of health and/or sickness. Additionally, the healthcare sector is often a major employer for cities and regions, allowing those who are called to it and those in allied professions a centralized place to attend to the wellness needs of the public. Whether a laboratory technician, nurse, physician, or transporter, healthcare facilities

DOI: 10.4324/9781003414902-9

offer its employees the ability and opportunity to influence the health and lives of their communities. The design of healthcare facilities should consider the different lenses through which employees engage in their work, including how spaces and equipment are situated around them.

The stories of relief, hope, and even what many may label as miracles are captured in the bricks and mortar of a neighborhood, community, and/or metropolitan healthcare facility. Connected to the physical structures and design strategies of these facilities are pieces of legislation, community funders, corporate businesses, and healthcare partners; they all share a vision for high-quality healthcare services that bolster communities.

Assuredly, healthcare facilities hold so much more than medical equipment and signage that demonstrate access to an elevator or a specific floor. The walls of these facilities also contain the critical conversations of those who periodically occupy the patient rooms, allow for the clinical updates to be delivered to anxious patients and their loved ones, and surround the spaces that support the families occupying the waiting areas.

The healthcare providers and professionals within these healthcare facilities, who scurry across the floors offering direction and providing the necessary healthcare services, spend much of their time in these facilities. These individuals and the people they serve deserve well-designed healthcare facilities that support their everyday tasks and activities of health professionals. This chapter will outline the importance of cultivating an inclusive and considerate experience through the design of healthcare facilities.

Promoting Health Equity in Healthcare Facilities

When considering best practices for effective healthcare settings, the concept of health equity often arises. Health equity refers to the assurance that everyone receives an optimal experience and has uninterrupted access to health services (Braveman, 2022). This goes beyond spatial understanding of accessibility, ensuring that access to health care is adequate and universally attainable. Consequently, when individuals speak of health inequities, they will often describe limited, stigmatizing, or unfair access points that are unnecessarily placed within a system (Braveman, 2022; Braveman et al., 2017). When considering this concept, it is important to understand the many factors or determinants influencing and/or shaping inequities within any given social, economic, or manufactured system. These considerations include the social determinants of health, describing how where one lives, loves, works, or plays affects overall health (Ataguba & Ataguba, 2020). These factors are frequently impacted by financial allocations, neighborhoods and the built environment, and oftentimes, policy decisions (Douglas et al., 2019). The existence of these determinants in any given setting (i.e., income, education, racial, gender), ensure that those who are privileged, with more direct access points to healthcare, encounter better health outcomes. These outcomes, taking place in physical and social settings, can manifest in a variety of ways, including through the onset or spread of disease, physical ability, and mental strife (Artiga et al., 2020).

The recognition of some of these privileges and access points became more apparent during the COVID-19 pandemic, often occurring in health-care spaces. During calls to action, not only was there concern for distancing and spacing, but the pandemic forced hospital administrators, clinic directors, and healthcare organizations to understand the acute and spatial challenges related to the spread of the virus. Since the rate of transmission was not yet understood, local and federal mandates to manage and control the spread of infection were enacted and updated in real time as more information became known. In the initial stages of the pandemic, the need for healthcare access and safety was thwarted by spacing and distancing requirements to limit the spread of infection. No longer were there open waiting rooms that could support dozens of sick patients and their families, nor were there open break rooms for clinical discussions of educational sectors over lunch. Areas where families could gather to sit and wait for results or updates regarding their loved ones were closed to the public. It was a time of strategizing and transforming the ways in which physical environments provided for equity, placement, and access.

Journalist Charles Blow wrote an opinion piece that spoke to the privilege of social distancing during the pandemic, revealing not only the challenge presented by the pandemic within homes and places of employment but also how practices within healthcare facilities were shaped by this new idea of creating space, safety, and effective treatment for patients (Blow, 2020; Keller et al., 2021). The pandemic evoked fear and anxiety among the public, placing stress on healthcare workers, administration, and city/public health officials. There became a larger issue within healthcare facilities concerning not only how to effectively treat patients while protecting their employees but also how to provide equitable treatment plans, patterns, spacing requirements, and the efficient execution of priorities (Nguyen et al., 2023).

Spacing usage and concerns throughout healthcare facilities during the pandemic were ad hoc, requiring creativity to meet the guidelines and rules put forth by the Centers for Disease Control and Prevention (CDC) and Offices of Public Health (OPH). At the outset of the pandemic, immediate action was needed to prevent further spread of infection; therefore, temporary paper signs were used to implement and convey changes to patient and wait protocols and processes for entering into the appropriate healthcare facilities and units. Chairs were utilized as barriers to block off sections of facilities, with caution tape and laminated signage strategically placed to separate and maintain appropriate distances. Once it was understood that the pandemic would be around for a while, signage became much more aesthetically pleasing. Stickers were placed on the floors to denote where individuals should stand in line, and signage was placed in accessible places to ensure that all individuals could see them. In hindsight, regard for language and cultural barriers was minimal and could have been further considered; more translingual signage, icons, and imagery would have been helpful for persons with visual, literacy, and/or comprehension concerns.

The digital divide was also illuminated during the COVID-19 pandemic. Challenges related to accessing telemedicine and the need to find ways to resolve them continued to be a problem for certain populations and geographical areas. Both patients and healthcare providers have faced challenges in establishing a seamless connection, and the delivery of technology and its target recipients remains a source of strain (Lopez de Coca et al., 2022; Reddy et al., 2022). The integrative use of technology has made it easier for healthcare spaces to deliver information and receive critical updates and assistance with treatment options and care. But should this only occur within the facility? In spaces where there are many diverse types of learners, spontaneous and unique challenges may arise that a digital connection may not be able to solve. The healthcare space can provide a quiet area, a comfortable seating arrangement, and even all the upgraded computer equipment necessary for a seamless and uninterrupted flow of virtual communication. But it is important to ensure that all patients and consumers who need that information can connect on the other end of the technological platform.

Perceptions of Equity in Healthcare Spaces

Perception can often override what some might consider truth because it frames the truth within the varied experiences of individuals. What is true for one individual in any given space may not be true for others. For instance, a patient or visitor who walks into a healthcare facility may feel that the entrance and signage are quite accessible; however, if the patient or visitor is in a wheelchair and has a visual impairment, they may feel the opposite. The presence of a reception desk just beyond the front entrance or even a coffee shop/station within waiting areas can indicate a variety of messages about a healthcare facility to its patrons, including but not limited to feelings of welcome and comfort, wait times for patients, staffing needs, and the ability to navigate through the facility itself.

Individuals may use their positive experiences at other healthcare facilities as a benchmark for all of them, leading to the perception that the ones that are different are less inclusive. Individual perceptions can shape how healthcare facilities are distinguished among their patrons in terms of reputation and quality of care. What an individual understands and feels in each can be quite different, shaping individual understandings of what is considered the best and most efficient patient care. Although many of these aspects may have nothing to do with the actual care of the patient, the experience one has accessing the facility can influence their perceptions of the quality of care they received.

Perception is often influenced by the bias that an individual carries. It can become the conversation that drives and steers how an individual responds and reacts to certain things. While hospitals and other healthcare facilities may have best practices for how they operate, there is not a standard roadmap or document that guides designers in how healthcare spaces and their subsequent equipment, furniture, signage, etc., should be located to make the greatest impact. It is often up to the discretion of the medical systems, city/district planners, and administrators on how to design healthcare spaces that are inviting and accepting to the public. These issues can be difficult to address in existing facilities, particularly when the original design of the building is not conducive to the creation of these spaces. Hence the importance of including designers and planners in the creation of healthcare facilities in various communities.

Spatial Considerations for Healthcare Facilities

It is understood by the general public that healthcare spaces are designed to facilitate and administer healthcare services to the public for a variety of healthcare issues. What is not as widely discussed, however, is that these facilities and their design also facilitate ancillary and auxiliary activities related to healthcare. These activities are just as important as the general care that takes place in healthcare facilities, and they should be equally acknowledged and considered during the design process. Ensuring that there is adequate spatial allocation and arrangements for teaching, learning, consulting, administrative, and maintenance tasks can improve the efficiency of healthcare delivery.

Teaching Spaces

Healthcare spaces have become flexible and adaptable based on the varied functions and roles of healthcare. What should not go unnoticed is the amount of education that is conducted in various healthcare spaces and agencies. A significant number of clinical professional students occupy healthcare spaces for certification, licensure, and/or internship. Educating students within their different disciplines and educating patients for continued health is yet another aspect of healthcare needs that should be considered.

As a training ground for various healthcare professionals, healthcare facilities are constructed and reconstructed based on need and regional and federal guidelines that are constantly being examined. Hospitals that support graduate and undergraduate medical programs, called major teaching hospitals, provide communities with services and clinical care that are more expansive than those that do not support teaching/medical education (Fisher, 2019). These hospitals represent approximately 5% of all hospitals in the United States (Fisher, 2019), but they can be the best spaces to test equity with the newest generations of healthcare profession learners. Hospitals that are granted the good fortune of supporting graduate medical education have institutional requirements that dictate the resources and infrastructure to support students, residents, and fellows. These requirements are revised every few years after changes within the healthcare arena and the unique needs of teaching adult learners (Accreditation Council for Graduate Medical Education [ACGME], 2022). The integration of learners such as medical students, nurses, physicians, and therapists and the various requirements necessary to provide an equitable teaching and learning environment are prescriptive in documents and even in competitive floor plans. For example, the Accreditation Council for Graduate Medical Education (ACGME), the organization that sets the requirements and standards for training and preparing medical residents in training, has an entire section of its institutional (healthcare spaces) requirements that is titled: *The Learning and Working Environment*. Within this section, it prescribes the necessary accessibility components and measures that a healthcare space must have to provide a safe, equitable, and healthy learning environment for residents and fellows in training (ACGME, 2022).

In academic teaching spaces, the requirements for the institutions that sponsor medical training to residents and fellows state "clean and private facilities for lactation with proximity appropriate for safe patient care, and clean and safe refrigeration resources for the storage of breast milk" (ACGME Institutional Requirements, effective July 1, 2022, III.B.7.d).(4), pg. 12). As the requirements continue, there is significant attention placed on the proximity and location of these spaces within the healthcare facility, giving the agency the nudge to consider the foot traffic necessary in certain areas to support individuals and provide optimal care. The institution must recognize not only the type of work that is happening in many different areas of the facility but also the employees' personal needs that are to be considered. Supporting the life choices and needs of employees and the varied types of learners that occupy the healthcare space is not just a choice anymore, but a requirement that agencies are placing at the hands of administration.

It is important to teach learners within the medical/clinical education system in spaces that are equitable, which includes their practice sites within each healthcare facility. If there are no equitable resources from facility to facility, it is the responsibility of the professional school or healthcare facility to provide adequate and reasonable support. If the professional school offers a specific type of provision for a student, the supporting sites that are affiliated with that institution should have similar supports on hand. The amount and structure of the resources, including spaces provided, need not be the same, but they should be consistent in opportunity and access.

Adequate resources and spaces can be difficult to come by due to distinct differences in the type of learning environment, location, the complement of administrative personnel, and the job or skill specificity within a particular profession. Additionally, administration or management's feelings about equitable resources and needs from facility to facility can also detract from the need to create similar experiences.

CASE STUDY

There are groups that occupy healthcare spaces who don't fit neatly into the categories of patient, healthcare professional, or staff member. One such group is medical residents and fellows. Medical residents and fellows engage with healthcare spaces in a way that gives them a very unique experience, falling somewhere between healthcare professional and student. Considerations for the medical student experience in healthcare facilities are just as important as those for the aforementioned groups if we are to create sustainable and resilient healthcare systems that maintain the health of populations over time. The following case study frames this consideration explicitly to demonstrate to healthcare professionals, designers, and planners the importance of keeping everyone in mind when making design decisions for healthcare facilities.

BACKGROUND

The ACGME sets all requirements for supporting the training of residents and fellows. The institutional requirements set by the ACGME articulate how educational environments, curricula, and physician faculty and staff are to provide support for a balanced and appropriate residency/fellowship. The healthcare agency, called the sponsoring institution, is responsible for ensuring that it has all the necessary financial, educational, clinical, and administrative support and resources to provide an appropriate training ground for the learners. ACGME's most recent requirements discuss the healthcare agencies' considerations on well-being, stating that the sponsoring institution must provide "sleep/rest facilities that are safe, quiet, clean, and private, and that must be available and accessible for residents/fellows, with proximity appropriate for safe patient care" (ACGME, 2022). There is no description about what this looks like for each institution, as the ACGME understands that there are a variety of different resources and spaces provided for graduate medical education across different healthcare facilities. Within the discussion of sleep and rest, however, it is understood that the agency should provide the necessary location and support for fatigue mitigation from the clinical and educational work that the residents and fellows perform within the healthcare space.

CASE

A few years ago, the author had a workshop with a hospital system. The day was filled with meetings with different administrators and healthcare professionals to discuss policy and healthcare practices. The organization arranged visits to various physician practices and laboratories as well as two of the hospitals within their health system. In a quick glance from the outside of each of the facilities, it was difficult to distinguish any huge difference between the two hospitals. Both facilities were similarly painted in their facades, with complementary landscaping and directional signage that was clear and visible.

When viewing the areas designated as sleeping spaces for residents and fellows at each facility, however, there were obvious differences. Facility A was located outside of the main hospital building, and though access was provided, the structure was not connected to the main hospital intercom system and was away from sound and interruption. This facility had modern furniture in the "living" space; a neat and well-stocked kitchen with food and snacks; and each sleep room had a wooden bed with a soft mattress, a thick well-maintained quilt, and a lamp with soft lighting. The sleeping space in facility A was separated from the living space and closed off by two large doors. The other hospital, facility B, had sleeping space on one of the hospital floors and was subject to loud overhead hospital pages via the intercom system. The entrance doors of facility B were automatic, with the steel doors creating a loud noise when they opened. Similarly to facility A, there was access to food and snacks within the sleeping space, but because of the foot traffic to partake of them throughout the day, trash and leftover food boxes accumulated, causing quite the distraction. The sleeping spaces in facility B opened to part of the living space; there was no divide between this public area, the living space, and the sleeping space. Beds in facility B were not as sturdy as those in facility A, and the quilts appeared a bit worn. Since it was on the floor of the hospital, the sleeping space was illuminated by fluorescent lighting and looked very similar to a pod of patient rooms.

There are several issues of note in this case study. One is that resource allocation and financial investment are important for ensuring the needs within any given agency are met. A lack of funding or a lack of dedicated intentional space to an area or specific program can be the difference between what employees, vendors, or patients may describe as equitable or inequitable. Here again is where the perception of what is imbalanced or different becomes apparent. This perception creates a feeling in the occupants that what should be afforded to all somehow isn't and possibly sends a greater message about how groups are valued or considered, even within the same hospital system.

Equipment Considerations in Learning Spaces

Healthcare spaces are educational settings that accommodate a diverse group of learners. As these individuals are being prepared to provide healthcare, the arrangement of their lecture or debriefing space can determine whether they think and feel included among the group. For these learners, teaching often includes discussions taking place around the bed of patients in real time. The spaces are often used to build trust and a relational type of interaction as the instructor positions himself or herself in a place where the information to both the patient and the learner is clearly understood. As learners typically stand around the patient's bed, it can pose challenges for those who have mobility issues and are required to stand for extended periods of time. In these cases, learners may have the desire to lean against furniture in the room, or even find a place to sit. However, the learner may avoid this if they think that their actions could convey indifference to their instructor, peers, and/or patients. In situations such as this, it is important for agencies to understand the limitations or participation restrictions of individual learners and ensure that healthcare spaces can accommodate their unique needs. Asking learners about special accommodations before the start of their program of study can build strong and trusting relationships among healthcare teams while also creating an inclusive and welcoming environment for everyone, including patients.

Designated rooms for didactic learning or clinical debriefing become very important when bringing together diverse individuals who manage the healthcare of communities. When considering the needs of all, it is important to remember that the goal of the room should be to hold and host individuals who share in the care of patients. Therefore, the actual layout and the equipment within the room should be considered.

Conference rooms, independent study rooms, and even meeting spaces should have appropriate and equitable considerations to the different types of learners and educational styles. It would be helpful if tables that are used in teaching rooms could be nested against each other. This makes it easier for storage and accommodations for seating distances and aisle width. Additionally, having tables with wheels that can be locked will aid with ease of movement during room configuration and for safety of the users. Prior to easy-to-store and -roll tables, these items had to be folded, often with the help of a couple of people, and were heavy and very awkward to move. With the more updated table designs utilized today, there is minimal delay and effort if a speaker or teacher wants to change the design of a room to accommodate individuals with different needs. These types of furniture considerations are helpful in all learning circles.

Not only are equipment needs and spatial arrangements a huge consideration, but the acoustics and delivery of sound can affect the engagement of those within the room and affect those with hearing impairments. There are many different aids to assist in enhancing sound. For example, larger conference rooms or auditoriums have dropped microphones that hang from the ceiling. However, there are throwable, wireless microphone systems that come in varied shapes, replacing the traditional handheld microphone. The presentation or lecture is transformed into a more engaging discussion, as participants can pass or toss this microphone system (shaped like a ball or cube) while having more dynamic interactions with participants. These types of enhancements disrupt systems of eye placement, keeping the focus on the individual who is in possession of the throwable system, and create more inclusive engagement for the participants. These considerations create a stimulating academic space that encourages preparation and interaction.

Hardware Solutions in Inclusive Healthcare

Hardware for doors, windows, and cabinets are typically eye-catching but they have a useful and functional purpose. The accessibility and ease at which the handles, knobs, or levers are positioned should be included in their design. In a recent visit to a hospital, the author observed that the food storage cabinets that contained snacks for physicians and residents were located above the sink and they did not have knobs or handles. There should be considerations for individuals who have height challenges or who have difficulty grabbing the underside of the cabinet. Access to places that hold food, drink, and other essentials should be easily accessible and safe.

While speaking of height challenges or restrictions of individuals in positioning food or even equipment, hardware on doors can also create challenges in equity. There are federal requirements and universal designs for doors in medical settings considering the latches, hinges, and even keys necessary for optimal safety (The Joint Commission, Clinical Impact. LS.02.01.10). In instances where the door handles and the positioning of hardware on doors or entry ways require persons to be a specific height to utilize them, accessibility challenges arise, and this can be harmful in health facilities where people need immediate access. It may be worth the investment to spend money on hardware that is universally designed for individuals at any height or ability level. Vertical door handles that extend the length of the door allow persons of any height to be able to access the door handle and pull it open for entry. There should also be a thought about how individuals who cannot adequately grip handles and those in wheelchairs will enter the spaces without difficulty. For example, some building entrances have a push button on the wall where the doors open automatically, making it easy for any individual to enter a particular wing or unit, no matter the individual's ability or stature. However, these may not be located at each major entry point or positioned in a place that is identified as needing an automatic opening option. Entrances and entry ways into clinics or any space therein should also consider size of equipment for patient transport as well as how employees can access the space, given any additional support that accompanies them. For example, some entrances into hospitals or clinics have one door that opens into the building, a short (approximately three foot) "landing," and then another door that is to be pushed open as well. Once the second door is pushed open, individuals are inside of the building.

For individuals with mobility issues, it would be very cumbersome to push open the first door, figure out how to hold that door, and then push the next door to enter the building. This becomes challenging for patient transporters who move patients through healthcare spaces in wheelchairs, as well as for individuals whose ability may be temporarily restricted by crutches, canes, or even an arm sling.

Challenges from site to site, even within the same healthcare system, can vary, and it is incumbent upon the host facility to understand the needs of its employees, learners, and/or patients within the setting. Oftentimes, that is accomplished by a simple question: *What do you need?*

Comfort Enhancements in Healthcare Spaces

As the design of healthcare facilities has evolved over time, there continues to be significant attention to improving health outcomes and the types of spaces that are included. Additional spaces include healing gardens, designated break rooms for employees, gift shops, canteens or cafeterias, and reflection rooms. They should be designed to accommodate both patients and employees in a way that can offer some relief and mind-body-spirit connection during the day.

Therapeutic Gardens

Healing gardens or indoor and outdoor spaces that tend to bring in nature and water have been constructed in many healthcare facilities. They address the mental, emotional, and social needs of any group of individuals while providing different design elements to heighten the senses in a positive way (Di Sivo & Balducci, 2019). The location of these spaces within the facilities' design and how patients, visitors, and/or employees are able to access these areas matters. Some of these gardens or therapeutic areas are much more elaborate in comparison to others, which may be due to a number of reasons. The goal of these spaces should be to ensure ease of accessibility and availability to everyone. Besides, what group of people do not want to have a positive experience when in a healthcare facility?

Reflection Spaces

Healthcare spaces often have places designated for prayer or meditation. These spaces are usually called multifaith spaces, as they do not usually ascribe to a particular religion or sect. These areas should be designated by signage that is highly visible, and staff should be aware of their location so they can direct individuals to them. Multifaith spaces avoid the distinction of religious or spiritual practices and lack symbols that may hint at a particular religious group. These spaces usually make use of natural materials like wood, include greenery, and use light explicitly to highlight important versatile spaces like altars and prayer areas. They should also be quiet and contemplative, so their location is especially important during the planning process. Signage should be easily noted, and the design of the space should be amenable to both patients and visitors, with special attention given to the spacing of elements, furniture, and how people with differing abilities navigate the space.

Lactation Spaces

Over the last few years, healthcare facilities have been more intentional about creating lactation spaces and lounges for their patients and employees. Corporate businesses, public administration facilities, and even colleges and universities now understand that it is important and in their best interest to create spaces that support mothers from a variety of backgrounds and abilities.

Lactation spaces are typically outfitted with comfortable seating, a mirror, accessible electrical outlets, a table, and some even have additional auditory and lighting features that can be controlled through a smartphone or device application. Occasionally, healthcare facilities provide basic equipment along with sanitation supplies so that individuals can clean their breast pump or wipe their hands/equipment after use.

The presence of lactation spaces in healthcare facilities should be communicated at various points along the main paths of travel and in waiting areas, and should also be in a manner that is inviting and supportive. Avoid taping signs since they appear temporary and could be perceived as a lack of commitment to supporting patients, visitors, or their employees. The appearance and position of signage may have individuals question the investment in the initiative and the importance of those who need and use the space. Similar to gardens and greenspaces, employees should be aware of the location of lactation spaces, as this increases the perception of commitment by the healthcare facility.

While there may be a need to lock these spaces or to have a sign-up process for their equitable use, the ability for individuals to access these spaces should not be met with difficulty or a lengthy wait time. Healthcare planning teams should consider not only the most ideal location of these facilities but also how many are needed for the size and occupancy of the facility. For example, a healthcare space that primarily services women and children may require a larger number of lactation spaces due to the population they primarily serve.

The interior design of these spaces should have soft, neutral color palettes that are calm and fixtures that can be used by anyone. Seating should be amenable to all body types and movable so that individuals can shape the environment to their needs. If an individual has physical challenges or uses assistive technologies and these considerations are not made in the design of a lactation space, it may prove difficult for certain individuals to enter these spaces. We must remember that motherhood is not the same experience for all individuals and that one's ability may often intersect with nursing mothers in interesting ways. Consideration should be given to those who have walking aids, assistance devices, or other challenges that may prohibit or limit access to this private and safe area for expressing breast milk.

The Value of Healthcare Planning Teams

Healthcare facilities should consider the following best practices when designing spaces that are accessible to/for all: First, signage should be easily identified, include elements such as braille, and should clearly announce who is allowed to enter the spaces. Second, there should be consistency in the names of units/spaces, and these spaces should be referred to in the same way by everyone throughout the facility. Educating employees about how these spaces should be termed allows everyone to feel that they are receiving "the same" information as others. When areas are referred to differently within a system, it creates discord and creates a question of why information is different to some. Many of these therapeutic spaces are learned about through interpersonal discussions and interactions and may even be portrayed on a hospital's website, highlighting the amenities of that healthcare facility.

Some of these spaces may contain elaborate fixtures and meticulous landscape, while others may only have the resources and funding to offer a disconnect from the work to enjoy fresh air or a change of scenery. No matter the value and detail that are placed on these spaces, what is important is their accessibility and usability. Healthcare planning teams should also consider if these spaces welcome and invite all individuals, regardless of mobility or physical/mental need and the maintenance needed to ensure continuous access.

There are so many unique spaces within healthcare facilities. The signage for these spaces should not only clearly communicate information to users but should also add to the healthcare facility's unique aesthetic. They should also contain identifiable signage that may include special awareness as well. No matter the orientation or type of a particular space or amenity of that space, the notification of what is available and where it is located is key. How a clinical space communicates to its patients, employees, and/or visitors that certain amenities are available and how to locate those amenities eases the anxiety of users, thereby minimizing the burden placed on staff to direct people through the facility.

Another important consideration is the outside of healthcare facilities. There are several variations in how this is done across healthcare facilities, with some being strategically placed around art or gathering fountains. Some seating areas have dynamic lighting that can be solar powered, and others are located among intentionally designed, highly manicured areas. Lighting is also an important consideration for healthcare facilities, with tall lights adequately positioned in parking areas and additional lighting at entrances to ensure the safety of visitors.

The differences in how this is done across different healthcare facilities depend on a variety of factors, including but not limited to financial investment, budget allocations, and the importance given to these features during the design and planning process. What is clear, however, is that the design and arrangement of these features can shape visitors' perceptions about the importance of their safety. Some visitors may speculate about the reasons more attention and funding were allocated to some features and not others. As a note, each of these considerations are speculative and contextual; therefore, healthcare planning teams should engage in extensive discussion about how these aspects should be addressed within their given institution, how they are associated with the quality of care, and how the institution would like to convey the importance of equity in the healthcare experience they provide. These considerations are not a question of which system has better care and treatment for its patients, but a question of the value placed on equitable experiences for all patients. Perception can lead to a conjecture of what individuals qualify as fair and equitable, allowing for concern and, in some instances, doubt.

Conclusion

The decision about what happens within a healthcare facility/space, what services are offered, and what specialty care is housed within it has forced the patrons, clients, and patients to truly take a step back and wonder about representation. The pandemic unleashed a wealth of information and plausible realizations that were rooted in perception, truth, and despair. For some, there was no need to visit a fountain or a garden of flowers; there was only a need to have a space to dry their tears and wrestle with the struggle of complex decisions. What employees, contractors, or patients in need of care ultimately wanted was the collective power of many voices. Voices that were understood and could represent the challenges and needs of those who were hanging on by a thread and latching on to some bit of hope and faith. There was a need to have the same access as the next person. There was a desire to be heard, even when there was no breath left to speak and no hope to fuel the spirit through.

Now as that time has appeared in the rearview mirror, the pluralism of voices is just as, if not more, important. The words of humanity communicated just a few years ago, words of solidarity and the fervent desire that everyone would have the same resources, access, and opportunities as the next person, would be considered in whatever space is being created. Whether the space is a boardroom or surrounding sidewalks, the design of spaces matters in all healthcare facilities. These things especially matter to those who are walking into healthcare facilities and entrusting strangers with their care. No matter the needs of the patient and their family, the support should be there. Many conversations happen around new construction, renovation, or just "re-invention" projects, but do these conversations have a diversity of perspectives? Having a variety of ideas and thoughts about where things should be positioned, situated, and even how they should be represented is crucial to cultivating inclusive spaces in all healthcare facilities.

References

Accreditation Council for Graduate Medical Education (ACGME). (2022, July 1). *ACGME institutional requirements*. III.B.7.d. (4). p. 12. https://www.acgme.org/globalassets/pfassets/programrequirements/800_institutionalrequirements2022.pdf

Artiga, S., Orgera, K., & Pham, O. (2020, March). *Disparities in health and health care: Five key questions and answers – KFF*. Retrieved October 11, 2023, from https://files.kff.org/attachment/Issue-Brief-Disparities-in-Health-and-Health-Care-Five-Key-Questions-and-Answers

Ataguba, O. A., & Ataguba, J. E. (2020). Social determinants of health: The role of effective communication in the COVID-19 pandemic in developing countries. *Global Health Action*, 13(1), 1788263.

Blow, C. (2020, April 5). Social distancing is a privilege. *The New York Times*. www.nytimes.com/2020/04/05/opinion/coronavirus-social-distancing.html

Braveman, P. (2022). Defining health equity. *Journal of the National Medical Association*, 114(6), 593–600.

Braveman, P. A., Arkin, E., Orleans, T., Proctor, D., & Plough, A. (2017). *What is health equity? And what difference does a definition make?* Retrieved September 24, 2023, from https://nccdh.ca/resources/entry/what-is-health-equity-and-what-difference-does-a-definition-make

Di Sivo, M., & Balducci, C. (2019). Patient-centered care approach: Strategies for healing gardens. *Journal of Civil Engineering and Architecture*, 13(12), 740–751.

Douglas, M. D., Josiah Willock, R., Respress, E., Rollins, L., Tabor, D., Heiman, H. J., Hopkins, J., Dawes, D. E., & Holden, K. B. (2019). Applying a health equity lens to evaluate and inform policy. *Ethnicity & Disease*, 29(Suppl 2), 329.

Fisher, K. J. (2019). *Academic health centers save millions of lives.* Retrieved April 23, 2023, from www.aamc.org/news-insights/academic-health-centers-save-millions-lives#:~:text=In%20addition%2C%20major%20teaching%20hospitals,of%20all%20inpatient%20psychiatric%20beds

The Joint Commission. (n.d.). *General requirements – clinical impact. LS.02.01.10: Building and fire protection features are designed and maintained to minimize the effects of fire, smoke, and heat.* Retrieved April 23, 2023, from www.jointcommission.org/resources/the-physical-environment/general-requirements/clinical-impact/

Keller, S. C., Pau, S., Salinas, A. B., Oladapo-Shittu, O., Cosgrove, S. E., Lewis-Cherry, R., Vecchio-Pagan, B., Osei, P., Gurses, A. P., Rock, C., Sick-Samuels, A. C., & Centers for Disease Control and Prevention Epicenters Program. (2021). Barriers to physical distancing among healthcare workers on an academic hospital unit during the coronavirus disease 2019 (COVID-19) pandemic. *Infectious Control & Hospital Epidemiology*, 43(4), 474–480. https//doi.org/10.1017/ice.2021.154.

Lopez de Coca, T., Moreno, L., Alacreu, M., & Sebastian-Morello, M. (2022). Bridging the Generational digital divide in the healthcare environment. *Journal of Personalized Medicine*, 12(8), 1214.

Nguyen, O. T., Merlo, L. J., Meese, K. A., Turner, K., & Alishahi Tabriz, A. (2023). Anxiety and depression risk among healthcare workers during the COVID-19 pandemic: Findings from the US census household pulse survey. *Journal of General Internal Medicine*, 38(2), 558–561.

Reddy, H., Joshi, S., Joshi, A., Wagh, V., Joshi, S. H., & Wagh, V. (2022). A critical review of global digital divide and the role of technology in healthcare. *Cureus*, 14(9).

8

PLANNING AND DESIGN PRINCIPLES FOR HEALTHCARE SETTINGS AT THE REGIONAL, CITY OR TOWN, AND NEIGHBORHOOD SCALES

Angela A. Appiah and Beverly Ann Collins

Introduction

The planning and design of diverse healthcare spaces at the regional, city, town, and neighborhood scale is not only about physical space and location. There should also be considerations made for the services that are incorporated into the built environment around these spaces to meet the needs of the population, with the goal of establishing a sustainable healthcare system (UN-Habitat and World Health Organization [WHO], 2020). Healthcare settings provide patients, their families, and employees with spaces for healing and preventative care. These spaces should be safe and have the ability to serve diverse populations in numerous settings such as acute, ambulatory, skilled nursing, clinics, and long-term and short-term care. In today's world, healthcare settings are also embracing advancements in technology, taking on forms such as telehealth, in-home care, and additions to standard care

DOI: 10.4324/9781003414902-10

areas (Janevic et al., 2023). Healthcare facilities must consider the care trajectory from prevention to tertiary care, survivorship, palliative care, and end-of-life care.

Thus, to provide appropriate healthcare to all, it is important to have interdisciplinary planning teams that focus on population needs through the lenses of inclusiveness, equity, and proactive design, as well as processes that consider short- and long-term needs. These interdisciplinary teams should consider not only immediate needs but also scientific breakthroughs, historical events such as pandemics, the lifestyles of underserved populations, and access to services. When the goal is to provide inclusive healthcare for all, the community needs must be factored into the process.

Planning and Design Teams and Stakeholders

A variety of people and organizations should be included when comprehensively planning and designing healthcare spaces at all scales. These individuals include healthcare administrators, environmental service professionals, planners and designers, municipal leaders, nursing and other clinical and nonclinical professionals, members of the communities being served, and information technology experts (Center for Medicare and Medicaid Services [CMS] & U.S. Department of Health and Human Services, 2020). While this list is not exhaustive, the idea is that these teams should comprise a diverse group of persons who consider end users and understand the healthcare needs of the internal and external community across various scales. Their involvement in the planning and design process can contribute to the satisfaction of facilities' end users and clients. Discussions about infection control guidelines, accrediting body standards such as those established by The Joint Commission, and regulations and permits requirements provided by the Department of Health (DOH) should precede the planning and design process. The design of healthcare spaces without these insights can lead to important aspects regarding access to healthcare settings being left out of the final design, leading to barriers that could affect the health of entire populations.

Administration Commitment

Healthcare settings should reflect a commitment to providing expert care that is personalized for each person and accounts for the diverse needs of everyone who uses the facilities. Strategic planning and the establishment of goals that lead to healthy outcomes are fundamental to planning, designing, and implementing healthcare services. The purposes of these facilities and their intended usage are identified during early stages of the planning phase and processes; therefore, inclusion of the public and community from the very beginning is essential for the implementation of productive healthcare settings. It is also important to garner the input of the professionals that work in these settings, ensuring their voices are considered at all phases of the design, planning, and implementation process. This aspect is crucial to the development of sustainable healthcare systems that are equipped for the growth of communities.

Commitment from administrators responsible for these facilities/institutions is essential for sustainable development of healthcare settings. Resource allocations, which include personnel and equipment, as well as the consideration of community needs and collaboration with stakeholders in the community, can be instrumental to the success of these projects. The Robert Wood Johnson Foundation (RWJF) report on the culture of health (2018) states that a culture of health is sustainable when individuals, communities, and organizations prioritize all aspects when designing and building, factoring in considerations such as where people live, learn, work, and play. Creating a healthy, equitable community must include policies and programs addressing various community needs. It is important to consider geography, location, systems, resources, and stakeholders when seeking to create a setting that supports a culture of health excellence. Healthcare settings therefore must consider the integration of multiple systems, strengthening the coordination of care through the diverse perspectives of public, community, and population health; social services; treatments; and transition of care (RWJF, 2018).

Community Assessment

To be successful, planning for and designing healthcare settings must include considerations about the needs of the communities they plan to serve. Therefore an interdisciplinary community assessment team should focus on gathering and reviewing the appropriate data before any design decisions are made. The assessment carried out by these teams should include the following:

- Whether there is a need for the healthcare setting.
- Current community health trends as a baseline for measuring the success of established objectives.

- The types of healthcare settings needed and their offered services.
- A variety of clinical scenarios that can assist planning and design professionals.
- Current barriers to healthcare access and the populations affected.
- Existing healthcare spaces and simulation of care processes, procedures, and experiences.
- Gaps in healthcare provisions and services in the city, town, or region.

The healthcare setting's operating procedures should be reviewed for a designated period, with updates, evidence-based practices, and new research taking place every one to two years.

The World Health Organization [WHO] (2023) identifies qualifiers for fostering the sustainable planning and design of healthcare settings; these qualifiers are established through an overview of health as both an input and outcome in the planning and design of healthcare settings at the regional, city or town, and neighborhoods. For example, planning compact places must include a review of data and evidence of risk mitigation strategies for excessive density to prevent unwanted health outcomes. The setting's social and physical factors are impacted by the population's condition within the community where they live, learn, play, work, and grow. Therefore, planning and design must be carried out with diverse and socially inclusive insights of these settings. Finally, planning involves evaluating places that are connected and resilient to climate change and a variety of disasters (WHO, 2023). The planning and design of healthcare settings should also include vertical and horizontal integration and decision-making support tools that consider meeting the care of diverse populations. Additionally, zoning, territorial processes, and economic strategies should be incorporated into the planning and design of healthcare settings (WHO, 2023).

The plan's operations are conducted by a diverse group of inter-professionals, collaborating toward the common goal of creating the appropriate healthcare settings to meet patient needs. An operations manager or director should lead the development of the healthcare facility project and be included throughout the design and implementation process.

The operations lead usually provides a checklist, sets planning meetings, and assigns each essential member a task to complete in preparation for the implementation stage. This individual also collaborates with the design team to review and help gain the necessary approvals from the city, region, town, and neighborhood municipalities. Some of the basic planning and design tasks include:

- Community and stakeholders workshops in preparation for the inclusion of their voices and concerns in the design process.
- The definition of the scope of the project, timeline, responsibilities, and appropriate stakeholders.
- Determination of the scope of various healthcare setting, based upon the needs assessment.
- A review of codes, standards, jurisdictional guidelines, policies, procedures, and laws affecting the project.
- A determination of funding sources, the establishment of a project budget, and the need for phasing if funding and project goals do not align.
- An audit of existing and potential barriers throughout the design and implementation stages.
- A list of short- and long-term goals for the healthcare setting and intended outcomes.
- The development of a timeline for program planning, design, and implementation, as well as post-occupancy evaluation.
- Sustainable strategies for design of the healthcare setting and ensuring facility efficiency over time.
- Partnership with internal and external stakeholders to support the utilization of the facility long term; these stakeholders should include residents within the community, community organizations, and other municipal representatives (WHO, 2023).

The planning of healthcare services should also include the integration of the appropriate infrastructure for technology. Other logistical concerns include a review of potential unknown conditions and the existing infrastructure for the required services.

Community Engagement

The benefits of community engagement in the planning and design process are numerous. Emerging as a necessary process for improved design outcomes for communities in the 1960s, it is now a best practice utilized by design and planning teams with the goal of eliminating health inequities within the regions, towns, and cities. Community design increases community buy-in and participation while also allowing community members to convey their needs and important community connections they would like to preserve. The community engagement process is usually carried out by an advisory committee, whose charge would be to focus on improvements to overall community health, as well as the economy, infrastructure resilience, strategies for disease prevention, and the promotion of healthy living. This involves including health centers, ambulatory facilities, and urgent care areas in deliberations concerning healthcare needs and the evaluation of care processes through a system-driven approach. The information obtained from community members determined during the engagement process assists with the identification of key areas for action within the design and implementation phases of healthcare facilities.

Throughput

Throughput is an essential consideration in the planning process. The healthcare facility should not only address current issues and needs but also have a visionary and innovative approach toward future challenges. The productivity of healthcare space has increasingly become a major concern for organizations the world over, and strategies for throughput – the process by which patients receive the appropriate care and efficiently flow through the various healthcare processes – while varied, are focused on addressing the barriers hampering the flow of patients (Åhlin et al., 2022). These barriers can also be spatial, where the design of the facility creates difficulties in navigating the healthcare process. It is important that adequate consideration be given to the design of healthcare facilities, allowing for efficient flow from the moment the patient arrives at the healthcare facility to the moment of discharge (Mangum et al., 2021). In considering the future, design and planning teams should also ensure that healthcare facilities have the ability to expand their beds and departments for a projected 1 to 30 years (De Angelo, 2023). In the era of global healthcare and population health, privacy for healthcare professionals and users is also essential in planning and design.

Privacy, Dignity, and Respect

Ensuring the privacy, dignity, and respect of facility users can be as simple as implementing and providing a person-centered approach in the healthcare setting. For example, the formation of an advisory council of patients, their families/caregivers, and professionals who are working within the facilities can help identify points of vulnerability regarding patient privacy. Planning teams should ensure that patient transport between departments occurs in such a way that they do not come in contact with others within the healthcare setting, that transfer between departments is done in an efficient manner, and that privacy is maintained. For example, the emergency department, radiology department, operating rooms, and intensive care units can be in close proximity to each other since patients are often transferred between them (De Angelo, 2023). Additionally, patients can be separated from each other by, for example, using curtains if there are no doors or walls (De Angelo, 2023).

Access to Healthcare Services

According to the Centers for Disease Control and Prevention (CDC), social determinants of health/healthcare inequities contribute to a lack of participation in health care (CDC, 2022). How facilities and health systems decide on what services to provide can also impact concerns with health equity. Barriers to accessing healthcare services include low socioeconomic status, lack of insurance, transportation, child care, and ability to manage work and family obligations. For example, transportation plays a major role in hospital-setting utilization. There are various methods of transportation that the facility and team designing the setting must consider. Investing in the transportation infrastructure to support population care decreases the chances of patients not following the continuum of the care process (WHO, 2023).

Cultural humility, competency, and collaboration among facility users and clinical professionals are necessary for providing equitable access to healthcare, subsequently addressing inequities in prevention, health promotion, treatment, and transitions of care.

The social determinants of health and inequities caused by them can be decreased further with careful attention to community needs, resources, and community engagements. Healthcare facilities, whether in regional, urban, rural, or global contexts, should be considerate of the individuals; groups/communities; populations; and physical, social, and political environment when planning for comprehensively designed spaces that meet the needs of populations.

Smart Cities

Some of the principles to consider when developing and planning healthcare settings include principles such as building a healthy community/neighborhood that is walkable, street connectivity with safe and efficient infrastructure, mixed land use, and streamlined living design (Public Health England, 2017). These edicts are often cited as smart growth principles, which outlines livability principles put forth by the 2009 U.S. Department of Housing and Urban Development, the U.S. Department of Transportation, and the Environmental Protection Agency's Sustainable Communities Partnership.

The livability principles are:

- High-quality transit, walking, and bicycling opportunities.
- Healthy, safe, and walkable transit corridor neighborhoods.
- Vibrant and accessible community, cultural, and recreational opportunities.
- Accessible social and government services.
- Transit-accessible economic opportunities.
- Mixed-income housing near transit (this currently supports the social equity principle, which measures housing affordability and income diversity).

These principles play a crucial role in the development of smart cities. Planning and design principles for healthcare settings at the regional, city, town, and neighborhood scales, when aligned with smart growth principles, provide essential tools for access and collaboration between service lines and populations that utilize the services. The facility's proximity to other services such as laboratory, diagnostic, and pharmacy services is also important. Considerations for transportation, access to healthcare nodes, zoning, and proximity to other services are crucial for patient throughput, services rendered, and care processes provided by interdisciplinary healthcare teams.

Collaborations

When healthcare facilities and systems design and incorporate components that allow for collaboration with public health agencies, duplication of efforts can be avoided. This can lead to a decrease of waste or unused resources, more access to and utilization of resources for those who need them, and access to alternative facilities and systems facilitated by public health agencies. Productive outcomes may include collaboration with increased resources, consideration of care management, and achieving overall population health goals. Additionally, concerns such as redlining can be avoided when public health agencies and those managing health systems facilities collaborate on services. Public health agencies' partnerships with health facilities are not only within the design and implementation processes. Ongoing review regarding the sustainment of services impacts the sharing of information and collaboration to enhance health equity in communities and among diverse populations in a positive manner.

Another example of collaboration among agencies would be between private and government sectors such as federally qualified health centers, serving both rural and urban underserved communities to design, implement, and sustain spaces that consider the population's health outcomes. This collaborative body works to ensure that facility spaces consider education, advocacy, preventive health services, and culture, and include processes and programs that will contribute to reducing the burden of lack of access to resources for healthcare (Healthcare Design, 2013). Partnerships between public health agencies and healthcare systems can enhance existing programs through streamlining programs that can be duplicative or neglected concerns.

Collaborations can contribute to increase in grants, funding, and inclusive community needs assessment solutions and implementation plans. The spatial design of facilities for all sectors must include assessment on financial support systems for the sustainability of these programs, the upkeep of spaces designed to improve primary health care services, and the throughput within community programs and health systems.

Emergency Preparedness

Regarding emergency preparedness, healthcare facilities should build collaborative relationships with public health and emergency preparedness agencies, ensuring that they have a comprehensive emergency operations plan (Federal Emergency Management Agency [FEMA], 2023; The Joint Commission [JC], 2022). Collaboration may include full-scale or tabletop exercises/drills related to a community disaster (e.g., train wreck, natural disaster, or chemical leaks), precipitating a response by first responders (Federal Emergency Management Agency, Emergency Management [FEMA], 2018). These exercises are often designed by public agencies with participation from acute and long-term-care facilities, local and regional Offices of Emergency Management, law enforcement, emergency medical services, fire officials, and other agencies (FEMA, 2018). A facility may also involve first responders in drills such as active shooter response. Healthcare facilities should also develop mutual aid agreements to support each other in the event of an emergency.

A good example of this collaborative effort is the Urban Area Security Initiative (UASI) – a Department of Homeland Security program that provides grants to assist state, local, tribal, and territorial efforts in preventing, protecting against, mitigating, responding to, and recovering from acts of terrorism and other threats. These grants provide grantees with the resources required for implementation of the National Preparedness System and working toward the National Preparedness Goal of a secure and resilient nation, allowing emergency management programs to devote funding to the unique planning, organization, equipment, training, and exercise needs in high-density urban areas (Department of Homeland Security [DHS], 2022). Crucial concepts for emergency preparedness are outlined in Table 8.1 (Centers for Disease Control and Prevention & U.S. Department of Health and Human Services, 2018).

Table 8.1 Key Concepts

Equipment and supplies	• Maintenance, supplies, and monitoring Establishment of concrete workflows related to policies, procedures, and SOPs: • Adherence to safety guidelines. • Providing a standard of care for populations.
An environment of care	• Guidelines for specific healthcare setting requirements. • State and federal requirements for all institutions.
Human resource management	• Requirements that must be met before and during the operations of healthcare facilities.
Information security	• The confidentiality aspects of population care. • Security assessments considerations for facility operations. • Privacy and security laws and regulations around confidentiality, care consent, documentation, and record-keeping. • Secure forums to protect personal health information (PHI). • Policies and procedures are required to guide practitioners.
Clinical and operational policies	• Policies and practices, the importance of them, and how they should be implemented in all healthcare settings.
Staffing	• Necessary staffing to support the services. • Teams and facilities equipped for providing accessible, people-centered services. • Maintaining a continuum of care across the lifespan. • Considerations of staffing and services based on diverse measures such as size, demographics, acuity, and health needs of the population. • Adequate clinical and operational staffing to determine the mix of cases and provide all people with access to health services.
The accessible location and operation hours	• Considering the location and operational hours of facilities against a diverse review of care needs to address the social determinants of health.

(Continued)

Table 8.1 (Continued)

	• Health facility design demonstrates compliance with accessibility standards for live/work/play environments. • Review of barriers, including those that are physical, economic, spatial, and temporal, to address access and recovery. • Primary health services, continuum of care, and hospitalization services must all be considered during design, as they impact one other.
The financial aspects	• The financial aspects of operating healthcare facilities must be considered during the planning and implementation of the plan to avoid closures or a decrease in services. • Evaluation of the ways and means of paying for services, including government reimbursement, self-pay, philanthropy, unemployment, uninsured, and resource availability. • For-profit and not-for-profit facilities reviews.
Improvements	• Quality improvement (QI), assurance (QA), safety, and evidence-based practice initiatives for successful care processes. • Facilities arrangements to support the provision of the highest-quality care, ongoing assessment of appropriate utilization of services, and quality of the services provided by diverse clinical professionals. • Documentation of improvement and performance, allowing for the evaluation of services that might result in changes that improve health outcomes.
Conflict of interest	• Considerations of standards of operation that cover conduct, conflict of interest issues, and actions that govern facilities, including that of population service, staff, and affiliates.

Definitions

Accreditation: The action or process of official recognition as having a particular status or being qualified to perform a specific activity.

Centers for Disease Control and Prevention (CDC): The nation's leading science-based, data-driven service organization that protects the public's health. Provides domestic and international leadership, as well as laboratory and epidemiology expertise, to respond to and work toward eliminating disease and assist with disaster response.

Centers for Medicare and Medicaid Services (CMS): In the context of emergency/disaster preparedness, CMS is responsible for assuring that healthcare providers and suppliers participating in the Medicare and Medicaid programs meet applicable federal requirements.

Disaster: A sudden event, such as an accident or a natural catastrophe, that causes great damage or loss of life.

Emergency: A serious, unexpected, and often dangerous situation requiring immediate action.

Emergency operations/disaster plan: A plan for responding to a variety of potential hazards.

External disaster: Occurs at locations separate from the healthcare facility and may include events such as transportation incidents or industrial accidents.

Functional/physical exercise: A realistic simulated event acted out by participants to test an emergency response plan and procedures using the ICS.

Hazard vulnerability analysis (HVA) and risk assessment are systematic approaches to identifying hazards or risks that are most likely to impact a healthcare facility and the surrounding community. Conducting a risk assessment/HVA is also a requirement in the CMS.

Incident: An occurrence, natural or artificial, that necessitates a response to protect life or property.

Incident command system (ICS): A standardized approach to the command, control, and coordination of on-scene incident management that provides a common hierarchy within which personnel from multiple organizations can be effective.

Internal disasters: Events that occur within the walls of the healthcare facility itself and may include incidents such as a power outage, water disruption, or radiation exposure.

The Joint Commission (TJC): Requires all healthcare facilities to have an emergency operations/disaster plan as specified in the performance elements of its Environment of Care standards.

Conclusion

It is well established that strategies for locations that include visioning, preplanning, investment in healthcare systems, projections of warnings, and coordination involving diverse stakeholders are important for convenient and effective healthcare response methods (Sharifi & Khavarian-Garmsir, 2020). Therefore, attention to planning, design, implementation, and management of all aspects of the facility planning and design is essential to services that are provided for healthcare.

It is important to assess for health inequities within older healthcare facilities and prevent them in new ones. There are planning and design principles and best practices that can promote inclusion and address barriers in healthcare delivery designs. However, it is important to balance them with input from the communities through community involvement and ownership in the healthcare delivery designs. Therefore, establish processes in strategic planning that identify and link how the designing of facilities can contribute to reducing health inequities in regions, cities, and towns, such as lack of resources and healthcare.

References

Åhlin, P., Almström, P., & Wänström, C. (2022). When patients get stuck: A systematic literature review on throughput barriers in hospital-wide patient processes. *Health Policy, 126*(2), 87–98. https://doi.org/10.1016/j.healthpol.2021.12.002

Center for Disease Control and Prevention (CDC), & Office of Health Equity. (2022, July). *What is health equity?* Retrieved August 25, 2023, from www.cdc.gov/healthequity/whatis/index.html

Center for Medicare and Medicaid Services (CMS), & U.S. Department of Health and Human Services. (2020). (Rev. 200 02.21.20). *State operations manual appendix A – survey protocol, regulations and interpretive guidelines for hospitals.* Retrieved May 29, 2023, from www.cms.gov/Regulations-and-Guidance/Guidance/Manuals/downloads/som107ap_a_hospitals.pdf

Centers for Disease Control and Prevention, & U.S. Department of Health and Human Services. (2018). *Public health emergency preparedness and response capabilities: National standards for state, local, tribal, and territorial public health.* Retrieved May 27, 2023, from www.cdc.gov/orr/readiness/00_docs/CDC_PreparednesResponseCapabilities_October2018_Final_508.pdf

De Angelo, C. J. (2023). *Planning and design principles for healthcare settings at the regional, city or town, and neighborhood scales.* Retrieved March 3, 2023, from https://insights.omnia-health.com/management/guiding-principles-hospital-design-and-planning

Department of Homeland Security (DHS). (2022). *Homeland security presidential directive.* Retrieved May 12, 2023, from www.dhs.gov/publication/homeland-security-presidential-directive-5

Federal Emergency Management Agency (FEMA). (2023). *National incident management system* (3rd ed.). Section IIIB: Incident command system. U.S. Department of Homeland Security. Retrieved May 12, 2023, from www.fema.gov/sites/default/files/2020-07/fema_nims_doctrine-2017.pdf

Federal Emergency Management Agency, Emergency Management (FEMA). (2018). *Incident command system.* Retrieved May 1, 2023, from https://training.fema.gov

Healthcare Design. (2013, October 8). *Preparing community health centers for effective design development.* Retrieved August 5, 2023, from https://healthcaredesignmagazine.com/architecture/preparing-community-health-centers-effective-design-development/

Janevic, M. R., Murnane, E., Fillingim, R. B., Kerns, R. D., & Reid, M. C. (2023). Mapping the design space of technology-based solutions for better chronic pain care: Introducing the pain tech landscape. *Psychosomatic Medicine, 85*(7), 612–618. https://doi.org/10.1097/PSY.0000000000001200

The Joint Commission (JC). (2022). R3 *report: Requirement, rationale, reference. New and revised standards in emergency management.* Retrieved May 29, 2023, from www.jointcommission.org/-/media/tjc/documents/standards/r3-reports/final-r3-report-emergency-management.pdf

Mangum, C. D., Andam-Mejia, R. L., Hale, L. R., Mananquil, A., Fulcher, K. R., Hall, J. L., McDonald, L. A., Sjogren, K. N., Villalon, F. D., Mehta, A., Shomaker, K., Johnson, E. A., & Godambe, S. A. (2021). Use of lean healthcare to improve hospital throughput and reduce Los. *Pediatric Quality & Safety, 6*(5). https://doi.org/10.1097/pq9.0000000000000473

Public Health England. (2017). *Spatial planning for health: An evidence resource for planning and designing healthier places.* Retrieved April 5, 2023, from https://assets.publishing.service.gov.uk/government/uploads/system/uploads/attachment_data/file/729727/spatial_planning_for_health.pdf

Robert Wood Johnson Foundation. (2018). *Building a culture of health.* Robert Wood Johnson Foundation (RWJF). www.rand.org/well-being/community-health-and-environmental-policy/projects/culture-of-health.html

Sharifi, A., & Khavarian-Garmsir, A. R. (2020). The COVID-19 pandemic: Impacts on cities and major lessons for urban planning, design, and management. *The Science of the Total Environment, 749*, 142391. https://doi.org/10.1016/j.scitotenv.2020.142391

UN-Habitat and World Health Organization (WHO). (2020). *Integrating health in urban and territorial planning: A sourcebook.* Retrieved April 2023, from www.who.int/publications/i/item/9789240003170

World Health Organization (WHO). (2023). *Urban planning is crucial for better public health in cities.* Retrieved April 1, 2023, from www.who.int/news-room/feature-stories/detail/urban-planning-crucial-for-better-public-health-in-cities

CHAPTER 8 ALERT

ALEXANDER LAZARD

The appearance of a place carries significant weight in shaping the perceptions of its inhabitants and visitors. It reflects the quality of service the environment provides, ultimately influencing how people feel about the streets and public spaces they interact with daily. The presence of pedestrian crossing signals, street trees, and blue-green infrastructure, as well as their condition and accessibility, all convey a message to users, whether they are navigating by car or on foot. The presence of pedestrian lighting and clear paths for walking or cycling to healthcare facilities also plays a crucial role, while the lack of these features unfortunately reveals a story of poverty and limited resources in the area. Every decision regarding infrastructure and land use has the potential to either attract or deter people from public spaces and amenities that can enhance their quality of life. Regional development of an equitable healthcare network is critical to communicating how an area views the health of its population. Overlaying a transportation plan that accommodates users' movement through and around healthcare creates more opportunities for access. Following this, zoning[1] can be prescribed to present variety near these healthcare centers, delivering a legible and permeable environment.

The development of an easily accessible, comprehensive healthcare system is vital for promoting the overall health and well-being of residents. A key achievement will be the establishment of a solid transportation network that ensures residents at varying stages of abilities can easily travel to and from healthcare facilities. This includes the orientation of sites around reliable and accessible public transit. Furthermore, creating a variety of amenities around healthcare centers through zoning can significantly enhance the overall user experience. This can include the development of nearby restaurants, shops, and recreational facilities that provide convenience and entertainment for patients and their families. Such amenities also contribute to a well-organized and user-friendly healthcare environment for patients and healthcare professionals alike. By investing in these measures, regions can actively demonstrate a genuine commitment to the welfare of their local populations. This commitment involves ensuring that healthcare services are accessible to all, regardless of socioeconomic status, race, or ethnicity. A robust healthcare system is vital for fostering a healthy and thriving community. It enables individuals to access timely and effective healthcare services, leading to better health outcomes and improved quality of life.

It is imperative to design healthcare spaces in urban areas that are fair and considerate of the existing conditions, accommodating all modes of transportation, including pedestrians, bicycles, transit, and cars. Rather than only prioritizing business-as-usual transportation methods such as cars, cities, towns, and neighborhoods should focus on creating areas that encourage interaction and provide pedestrian pathways for unrestricted movement. This will promote overall health and well-being by encouraging physical activity and socialization. This also ensures that everyone can have equal access to quality healthcare and a high standard of living. Providing adequate pedestrian infrastructure, such as sidewalks, crosswalks, and bike lanes, can significantly enhance access to healthcare facilities. Similarly, the availability of green spaces and parks can improve residents' mental and physical health.

The physical appearance of public spaces plays a vital role in shaping the perceptions and experiences of its users, applying personalization to urban form, and converting areas you pass through to places you want to be nearby. Therefore, it is crucial to design and maintain public spaces that are safe, accessible, and aesthetically pleasing. Including public art and street furniture can create an inviting and attractive environment that encourages people to visit and interact with the space. The equitable design of healthcare spaces in urban areas should anticipate the context and adjust/rehabilitate critical paths to accommodate all modes of transportation, including pedestrians, bicycles, transit, and cars.

It is essential to recognize the impact of zoning and land use on living environments and how they can be utilized to promote equitable and inclusive healthcare settings. We must consider how people access services and facilities, what complementary uses can be incorporated, and how land use can contribute to rehabilitating economically disadvantaged or historically underserved areas. To improve the urban design of regional, city, or neighborhood healthcare nodes, it is essential to accommodate the needs of all users, foster viable economic uses, and promote a stronger sense of community and well-being in the surrounding blocks and parcels. This will create a more welcoming and inclusive environment for all individuals, regardless of their background or socioeconomic status. Ultimately, by prioritizing the needs of people and promoting social interaction and physical activity, we can create a more vibrant and healthy community.

ALERT – LAFAYETTE, LA

The individuals residing in Census Tracts 9 and 11 face several challenges as they strive to attract investments in their area. Based on data from the U.S. Census Business Builder, it has been found that a significant percentage of the residents in this area do not have access to a car, with 22.2% of the population falling into this category. Furthermore, a significant portion of the people – 39.1% – live in poverty, with an average income of $36,161. With these barriers in place, the residents of this area are facing significant challenges in accessing healthcare services that are both affordable and convenient.

While a health services center is available in the area, it closes at 5:30 p.m. (SWLA Center for Health Services, 2023), which is inconvenient for most residents who work during the day. While public transit is available at night, it takes nearly 50 minutes to reach the bus station to transfer to the emergency room. Additionally, the closest urgent care facility open after hours is located 4.2 miles away, and the nearest emergency room is 3.8 miles away. Unfortunately, access to these facilities requires many residents to traverse six-lane roads and an interstate system, making it extremely difficult for residents to commute safely by walking or biking.

This situation reveals the unfairness of regional, city, and town planning for equitable healthcare access. An area with a low rate of car-ownership should have accessible and safe healthcare options. As such, it is essential to consider the following questions in this situation:

1. How can we ensure that all residents have regional and local access to affordable and convenient healthcare options?
2. What steps can be taken to make healthcare services more accessible to those who do not have access to a car?
3. How can transportation and zoning be used to improve a resident's access to critical care?

By addressing these questions, we can work toward creating a more equitable and just community for all.

SWLA Center for Health Services. (2023, June 30). *Lafayette health clinic*. SWLA Center for Health Services. www.swlahealth.org/locations/lafayette/

Note

1 Zoning: The division of a city or county by legislative regulations into areas, or zones, which specify allowable uses for real property and size restrictions for buildings within these areas. Also, a program that implements policies of the general plan.

9

THE DESIGN OF HEALTHCARE CENTERS/HOSPITALS AND HEALTHCARE CAMPUSES

Twila Sterling-Guillory and Veronica D. Woodard

Introduction

Healthcare centers, hospitals, and healthcare campuses are different scales of physical healthcare environments (PHEs) that provide healthcare services to patients, their families, and the communities in which they are located. *Healthcare centers* are a collection of healthcare facilities, integrating and providing access to a number of healthcare services (Health Resources and Services Administration [HRSA], 2023). Their services are out of the scope of what hospitals provide, such as clinics, pharmacies, substance abuse and mental health services, and many more, all within close proximity to each other. The primary goal of this model is to address disparities in healthcare and provide a more coordinated healthcare experience for patients living within that geographic area. Thus, healthcare centers are patient-directed organizations that seek to remove cultural barriers to healthcare for a variety of different groups within a community (HRSA, 2023). On the other hand, *hospitals* are the most complex types of healthcare facilities (Ahmed et al., 2015). Healthcare facility is a broad term that can be used to describe several

DOI: 10.4324/9781003414902-11

building typologies whose primary function is to provide health services to patients. Four main categories of healthcare services and buildings fall within these facilities. The categories are primary or community, secondary, tertiary, and quaternary care. Facilities can range from small clinics to large complex hospitals (Ahmed et al., 2015). Finally, *healthcare campuses (health district or health village)* are large sites that contain a collection of facilities dedicated to both acute and ambulatory healthcare services, all under one healthcare or educational entity (Silvis, 2014). The facilities include hospitals, clinics, specialty medicine facilities, and even research centers. The facilities that make up healthcare campuses share infrastructure and are often interconnected in function (Silvis, 2014).

Most of the population in the world resides in an urban area, and there is a paradigm shift to placing PHEs within communities instead of on their outskirts and providing population wellness care instead of sick care (Silvis, 2014). Their services promote positive healthcare experiences, reduce disparities, and improve health outcomes for all. Additionally, their focus on wellness reduces healthcare costs (Congress for New Urbanism [CNU], n.d.). Unfortunately, an interruption in their services can have significant negative impacts on the health and well-being of the residents in the communities in which they are located. Therefore, the focus of this chapter includes the design considerations that are necessary to promote safe facilities for patients, staff, and their communities during adverse events such as emergencies and disasters.

Disasters are more detrimental to poor communities and developing countries (World Health Organization [WHO], 2015), and they have increased in number and severity within the past decade or two. Many hospitals are built without taking the occurrence of these adverse events into account. In addition, when maintenance is neglected, systems that are critical for the functioning of the hospital or PHEs deteriorate over time. It is important to design safe PHEs and improve the safety of those that are already in existence.

Safety Evaluation of Physical Healthcare Environments

The Hospital Safety Index is a tool that was designed to assess the safety of tertiary, university or major referral hospitals, but "it can be applied to the evaluation of other health facilities and can be used as a reference to evaluate other public services and facilities, subject to the corresponding technical adaptations being made and national and international standards being taken into account" (WHO, 2015, p. 12). Therefore, this tool can be used by PHEs to determine their vulnerability to adverse events such as emergencies and disasters. A limited overview of this tool will be discussed with emphasis on the evaluator and Forms 1 and 2.

Overview of the Hospital Safety Index

The Hospital Safety Index is an objective and standard tool that is used by evaluators to determine whether providers are able to provide safe healthcare services during and after a disaster or emergency (WHO, 2015). The assessment is expected to reveal strengths and opportunities for improvement to safety and prevent interruption of services. There is a section on methodology, two forms that should be completed, a section on the scoring systems and safety index, and a basic glossary of terminology.

The evaluator can use the methodology section to receive an "overview" and considerations during the completion of the checklist. The first form, "General information about the hospital" (Annex 1) [p. 12], is to completed by the PHE that is being evaluated, while the third form, "Safe Hospitals Checklist" (Annex 2) [p. 12], is to be completed by the team that is conducting the evaluation.

Form 1 − *General Information* requires the name and address of the health center, hospital, or healthcare campus. The name of the senior management and disaster or management staff, amount of personnel, beds, and occupancy rate in addition to a drawing of the facility and "surroundings." In addition to the hospital treatment and operating capacity which includes: amount of beds by specialty, such as medicine, intensive care, surgery, operating rooms, operations related to disaster and emergency, capacity to expand if there is an emergency/disaster, and nonclinical staff (WHO, 2015).

Form 2 − *Safe Hospitals Checklist* is a four-section list that consists of 151 items, rated as low, average, or high, that provide an initial assessment of how safe the PHE is and its ability to continue services if an adverse event occurs. The first section addresses hazards that affect its safety and its role in managing an event, and the second module addresses the structural integrity of the building and exposure to previous events. The third addresses nonstructural elements that are essential to their function and include office and laboratory equipment and critical systems such as electricity and water and protection from fire. The fourth module addresses the management of the disaster or emergency, including the plans that are in place to deal with the event (WHO, 2015). This limited discussion provides designers with some areas that they should focus on when designing new PHEs and renovating existing ones. The complete document can be accessed by readers who wish more information.

Design Considerations for Physical Healthcare Environments

There are some general design objectives for new and existing PHEs, some contributors to the goal of quality patient care, and some key to design. According to WHO (2015) the four design objectives that new and existing PHEs should adhere to are:

1. Ensure that services are uninterrupted during and after the adverse event.
2. Safety of patients, their families, and healthcare employees.
3. Protection of structural integrity, equipment, and critical systems such as electricity, water, and communication.
4. Resilience to future adverse events and climate changes.

Additionally, BluEnt (2022) states that designers should consider the location, the types of patients, their mission and vision, and the safety and productivity of employees with the goal of quality patient care. Furthermore, it is important to adhere to building codes and regulations and BluEnt (2022) *keys to design*. BluEnt suggests that designers focus on the expectations of patients and the needs of employees. Thus, the following design consideration/features should be incorporated in the design of PHEs:

• Front desk – A private space for front desk staff where patients feel welcomed, since making a positive first impression to patients and their families is important.
• Accessibility – Adhere to and exceed Americans with Disabilities Act requirements. For example, wide sidewalks and corridors that will allow two wheelchairs to pass beside each other.

- Wayfinding – Clear wayfinding so that patients, their families, and patrons can navigate the facility independently and easily.
- HVAC system – An effective heating, ventilation, and air conditioning (HVAC) system.
- Furnishings – Stain- and rust-resistant furnishings that are comfortable and can be cleaned easily.
- Patient focused – Rooms with single beds for one patient per room and with space for their families.
- A biophilic space – Spaces for patients, their families, and staff to obtain fresh air and sunlight and perform activities. These can be achieved by incorporating windows and gardens with walkways in designs.
- Emotional and spiritual needs – Dedicated spaces for everyone to meditate, pray, or have their spiritual needs met.
- Rest space for employees.
- Standard layout of each patient room and location of medical supplies – The former ensures that patient rooms are close to the nurses station so that they can be helped quickly, and the latter helps to reduce errors.

Structural Design Considerations

It is important to focus on the structural design of PHEs (Luke et al., 2021) and adhere to the specific standards that are required in building design. The development, promotion, and enforcement of these standards, along with the various approvals required by various departments within city, state, and federal government entities, all aid in designing buildings that are structurally safe.

A team of experts along with administrators and managers are needed to ensure that the PHEs are structurally sound. They should inspect the building sites and their surrounding areas to determine whether there are potential risks and mitigate them. A geotechnical engineer or one who specializes in seismic resistance has to be a team member if the site of a new build is in an area that is prone to earthquakes (WHO, 2015). Other team members include engineers who have expertise in structural engineering; architects who are trained in hospital design; specialists in disaster and emergency management, hospital critical systems, biomedical engineering and equipment, and/or electrical and mechanical maintenance; end users such as healthcare professionals such as physicians and nurses; and others such as security specialists (WHO, 2015). Designers can also use green practices and focus on communities by encouraging partnership between developers, public health, and stakeholders (Lindberg et al., 2021).

Conclusion

The health of thousands of people worldwide is affected by disasters (Luke et al., 2021). Therefore, when a disaster occurs, providing immediate healthcare services is imperative because of the potential negative impacts of a lack of healthcare services. Health centers, hospitals, and healthcare campuses need to be designed to be resilient to the impacts of adverse events. The Hospital Safety Index tool and the design considerations that were presented can assist administrators in achieving resilience.

References

Ahmed, T. M. F., Rajagopalan, P., & Fuller, R. (2015). A classification of healthcare facilities: Toward the development of energy performance benchmarks for day surgery centers in Australia. *HERD: Health Environments Research & Design Journal*, 8(4), 139–157.

BluEnt. (2022). *What you need to know about healthcare facility design*. Retrieved November 27, 2023, from www.bluentcad.com/blog/healthcare-facility-design/

Congress for New Urbanism. (n.d.). *Health districts: Our projects*. Retrieved November 27, 2023, from www.cnu.org/our-projects/health-districts

Health Resources and Services Administration. (2023, May). *What is a health center?* Retrieved October 1, 2023, from https://bphc.hrsa.gov/about-health-centers/what-health-center

Lindberg, R., Bever, E., & Millett, S. (2021, March 21). *How community development financing can help support healthier neighborhoods*. Retrieved August 11, 2023, from www.pewtrusts.org/en/research-and-analysis/articles/2021/03/01/how-community-development-financing-can-help-support-healthier-neighborhood

Luke, J., Franklin, R., Aitken, P., & Dyson, J. (2021). Safer hospital infrastructure assessments for socio-natural disaster – a scoping review. *Prehospital and Disaster Medicine*, 36(5), 627–635. https://doi.org/10.1017/S1049023X21000650

Silvis, J. (2014, April 21). *Designing for wellness: The healthcare campus of the future*. Retrieved October 11, 2023, from https://healthcaredesignmagazine.com/trends/architecture/designing-wellness-healthcare-campus-future/

World Health Organization. (2015). *Hospital safety index: Guide for evaluators* (2nd ed.). Retrieved November 27, 2023, from www.who.int/publications/i/item/9789241548984

CHAPTER 9 EXAMPLE

ALEXANDER LAZARD

Considerations regarding how people move inside and around buildings can dramatically contribute to equitable design. It can also create a unique differentiator across healthcare campuses. Building structures often reflect history, and material selections further personalize health centers and hospitals. By creating a network of walkable paths between buildings, parking structures, transit stops, and public spaces, the health campus can offer a comprehensive user experience with a variety of experience options. This approach accommodates users of all abilities, enhances their on-campus experience, and gives them greater access to health facilities. It also encourages physical activity and interaction with other users along the way. Overall, it promotes confidence in parking, walking, or biking.

To truly optimize the experience of healthcare campuses, it is essential to invest in what users experience as they get around. This means strategically placing amenities throughout the area, such as rest stops furnished with comfortable benches, convenient charging stations for electronic devices, bottle filling stations to encourage hydration, and even dog fountains for guests and service dogs. These rest stops should be in well-lit areas that are easily accessible at all times of the day so that users can enjoy the "payoffs" along their journey. By doing so, individuals will be incentivized to explore different services and facilities across the campus, ultimately increasing their overall engagement and satisfaction.

One considerable benefit of strategically placing amenities is that it can significantly reduce the perception of long distances between buildings or parking lots. When users have access to frequent rest stops along their journey, they are more likely to perceive the journey as manageable and enjoyable rather than overwhelming or exhausting. Additionally, placing these amenities between annexes can encourage connectivity, efficient movement, and exploration. By thoughtfully designing the campus layout to promote these aspects, healthcare facilities can create a more positive and memorable experience for their patients, visitors, and staff.

Schiller and Kenworthy (2018) discuss "permeability" in their writing, *An Introduction to Sustainable Transportation Policy, Planning and Implementation*. This term describes an interconnected path network that offers multiple direct ways through and around. The network of paths within a permeable area is exceptionally intricate, with each path cleverly interconnected in a manner that provides a multitude of options for navigation. The paths are thoughtfully designed to cater to different needs, with longer paths perfect for strolls and shorter routes for convenience and ease of access to healthcare services. The safety of every individual who uses these paths is of utmost importance and, as such, great care is taken to ensure that the paths are designed with increased visibility in mind. To further enhance safety, "casual surveillance" is implemented by strategically placing "windows and doors that face directly onto the paths, providing an additional layer of assurance and peace of mind for all who utilize it."

Additionally, pedestrian paths throughout a campus should contemplate the Americans with Disabilities Act (ADA) recommendations (U.S. Department of Justice Civil Rights Division, 2010). It is important that health campuses are accessible and inclusive of all users, regardless of their abilities. Relevant questions that ADA compliance addresses include:

- What does the ADA classify as accessible arrival points within a site?
- What does the ADA classify as accessible exterior routes within a site?
- What are the components and elements of accessible routes?
- What clearances should be observed along accessible routes?
- What are the minimum requirements for passing spaces along accessible routes?
- What are the curb ramps, and what function do they serve?
- What does Title II of the ADA require concerning curb ramps at pedestrian crossings?
- What are some critical characteristics of accessible curb ramps?
- What are some standard ramp designs?
- How can you tell if a curb ramp is accessible?
- What steps can you take to ensure your entity complies with the ADA requirements for accessible curb ramps at pedestrian crossings?

EXAMPLE – VIRGINIA BEACH, VA

Sentara Princess Anne Hospital is a well-known medical institution located in the southern part of Virginia Beach. Since its inception in 2011, the hospital has been a leading provider of top-notch healthcare services. The hospital's many benefits are breast care, cancer treatment, maternity care, neurosciences, and surgical procedures. To enhance their already impressive facilities, the hospital sought the expertise of American firm Vanasse Hangen Brustlin (VHB) to develop its master plan. The resulting project included a comprehensive landscape design tailored to promote pedestrian activity. The campus was designed with the needs of patients, visitors, and staff in mind, with the goal of providing a safe and comfortable environment for everyone. Thanks to the thoughtful and innovative design, the hospital can offer a unique and enjoyable experience to all who visit.

The plan includes the following:

- Surface parking designed to provide a seamless patient experience when accessing healthcare services and equipped with integrated walking paths that ensure easy and convenient access to medical center suites.
- Thoughtfully placed seating areas along the routes that connect buildings. These designated rest stops provide a convenient place for individuals to take a break and relax before continuing their way.
- An interconnected network consisting of several paths that can be used for multiple purposes and lead directly to various destinations.
- Visibility to common areas and paths via windows and doors, creating an environment that promotes transparency and accessibility.
- Connecting with public transportation to provide accessibility for individuals who depend on city services.
- ADA-compliant sidewalks with wheelchair-accessible paths and transitions. This ensures those with mobility issues can navigate sidewalks safely and comfortably without barriers or obstructions. (Vanasse Hangen Brustlin [VHB], 2023)

Sentara Princess Anne Health Campus has taken great care to ensure all their guests feel welcome and comfortable throughout their facilities. They have implemented a variety of equitable and inclusive practices that are evident in their outdoor spaces. From accessible entrances and pathways to public space amenities, every detail has been carefully considered to enhance the overall experience of their guests. The result is a safe and welcoming environment accessible to all, regardless of their needs or abilities. Consider the following questions in your assessment of this project:

1. What "payoffs" along the journey around the Sentara Princess Anne Health Campus were provided?
2. How is permeability demonstrated?
3. What additional services or features can be offered to improve the user's experience from building to building or lot to building?

References

Schiller, P. L., & Kenworthy, J. R. (2018). *An introduction to sustainable transportation policy, planning, and implementation.* Routledge, Taylor Francis Group.

U.S. Department of Justice Civil Rights Division. (2010). *Project civic access toolkit, chapter 6: Curb ramps and pedestrian crossings under title II of the ADA.* Archive.ADA.gov Homepage. Retrieved July 7, 2023, from https://archive.ada.gov/pcatoolkit/chap6toolkit.htm

Vanasse Hangen Brustlin. (2023). *Sentara Princess Anne health: Healthcare. VHB.* Retrieved July 7, 2023, from www.vhb.com/institutions/healthcare/sentara-princess-anne-health-campus/

10

CONSIDERATIONS FOR AMBULATORY SETTINGS

Harmony Rochon and Christian Wild

Introduction

Inclusive design as a pathway to increased health equity is an emerging field of study with limited research, yet it provides a clear lens for design and development that positively impacts accessibility and equity for general populations as well as for vulnerable and underrepresented communities (Lanteigne et al., n.d.). Inclusive design is defined as an approach for creating safe, equitable, and accommodating environments for a diverse set of users and has also expanded to address social justice, equity, and broader inclusivity (Lanteigne et al., n.d.). Researchers in this area have identified the Centers for Disease Control and Prevention's (CDC) social determinants of health as a useful framework for exploring inclusive design in the development of healthcare spaces that promote equity, access, and the foundations of a healthy life for diverse populations utilizing healthcare systems (Lanteigne et al., n.d.; Owusu-Ansah et al., 2023).

DOI: 10.4324/9781003414902-12

> The Centers for Disease Control and Prevention (CDC) defines social determinants of health (SDOH) as the nonmedical factors that influence health outcomes. They are the conditions in which people are born, grow, work, live, and age and the wider set of forces and systems shaping the conditions of daily life. These forces and systems include economic policies and systems, development agendas, social norms, social policies, racism, climate change, and political systems (Centers for Disease Control and Prevention, 2022, para 1).

The social determinants of health are identified within five domains: economic stability, education access and quality, healthcare access and quality, neighborhood and built environment, and social and community context (CDC, 2022). This chapter will focus on healthcare access and quality. Preliminary research suggests that review of healthcare facility layouts, emergency medical system functions, and patient-provider interactions through the lens of inclusive design will promote increased health equity (Lanteigne et al., n.d.). This can be achieved through *communication, assessment, the cultivation of user-friendly environments, and person-centered approaches*. Enhanced health communication occurs when there is clear messaging (verbal, written, visual signage) and services to patients including preadmission care, care within the healthcare center, and postadmission follow-up. Equally important is assessment, ensuring that health service providers are getting valuable feedback from patients, especially those in marginalized populations. Next is the cultivation of user-friendly environments, which requires designers to consider whether the built environment promotes well-being, has ease of access, and is socially inclusive of diverse populations of patients. Lastly, person-centered and patient-centered approaches are vital to increasing health equity, and inclusive design must consider all identities held by a patient in order to help healthcare providers understand, acknowledge, and treat the whole person (Lanteigne et al., n.d.). These approaches constantly ask what is best for the person/patient and how design can support healthcare environments for comfort and safety. Patient-centered design strategies include creating opportunities for quiet/stimulation, privacy/visibility, the addition of handrails, adjustable beds, and flooring that is shock absorbing (Piatkowski & Taylor, 2016).

Inclusive healthcare design also requires reflexive introspection among builders and the architects who are creating healthcare spaces. It is important to ask questions such as: Who is designing/building the facility or space? Are healthcare providers included in the design process? Have the voices of patient populations been included throughout the process via research and focus-group interactions? Have marginalized populations been included in the design process? It is critical that the design process be community-driven, including various stakeholders and perspectives to ensure inclusive design practices truly lead to greater health equity (Lanteigne et al., n.d.). Consideration of these various perspectives also highlights the need for balancing competing priorities when aiming for inclusive design and health equity. Sustainable design and green building are mainstream ideas within design communities, however, these two lenses do not guarantee inclusivity. The authors propose an overlapping paradigm that includes sustainable and green building encompassed within an inclusive design framework to highlight the holistic and overarching considerations made during the inclusive design process.

A scholarly consideration of inclusive design also requires review of the concepts of universal design and human factors design. Many frameworks view these labels as interchangeable, although there are some important nuances in each approach. Universal design and human factors design are subsidiary concepts under the inclusive design umbrella; however, they take a narrower approach that does not focus on broader social justice and equity issues. Human factors design takes the narrowest approach, focusing on the relevant design aspects necessary for healthcare providers and patients to have optimal experiences – specifically for providers to complete tasks in an efficient and safe environment and for patients to experience high levels of comfort. The goal is to optimize human performance and create an environment that suits the provider, patients, and tasks to be completed (Avery et al., 2015). Universal design is broader and is defined as "the design of products and environments to be usable by all people, at every changing level of need, to the greatest extent possible, without the need for adaptation or specialized design" (Piatkowski & Taylor, 2016, p. 5).

Piatkowski and Taylor (2016) outlined seven principles of universal design that are essential in the development of highly accessible environments. The adoption of universal design principles brings the design process closer to inclusive design and health equity. The seven principles are outlined in Table 10.1.

Table 10.1 The Principles of Universal Design

Principles	Definitions
Equitable	Useful and marketable to people with diverse abilities
Flexible	Accommodates a range of preferences and abilities
Simple and intuitive	Easy to understand for any user
Perceptible information	Communicates information effectively
Tolerance for error	Minimizes hazards and unintended actions
Low physical effort	Can be used efficiently and comfortably
Size and space	Appropriate for use regardless of the user's body size, posture, or mobility

As the field of inclusive design builds momentum, it is relevant to assess the overlaps and distinctions between human factors design, universal design, and inclusive design. The discussion questions that follow will assist with critical conversations about these concepts.

Discussion Questions

- Compare and contrast inclusive design, human factors design, and universal design. What are the similarities and differences?
- Does the use of human factors or universal design approaches guarantee inclusivity?
- Give examples of some inclusive design elements.

Inclusive Design for Out-of-Hospital Healthcare Settings
Ambulatory Care Centers

Out-of-hospital healthcare settings encompass clinics, mobile health facilities, ambulatory care centers, and emergency medical transportation. Inclusive design approaches and elements are equally important considering that millions of patients are treated annually in healthcare settings that are not within hospital walls. Current estimates show that 22.5 million procedures are performed in ambulatory surgery centers annually within the United States and that there are close to 6,000 Medicare-certified ambulatory centers operating in the United States (Ambulatory Surgery Center Association [ASCA], n.d.).

Ambulatory care centers have a vital role in healthcare systems. Hospital stays can be economically costly and can lead to negative patient outcomes, such as increased risk of complications, hospital-acquired infections, and slower recovery rates (Hamad & Connolly, 2018). Many patients, especially the elderly, recover quicker in environments that are safe, familiar, and comfortable (Rhode, 2021). Furthermore, well-designed ambulatory centers can alleviate the demand on inpatient hospital beds and reduce the likelihood of hospitals reaching capacity while providing the same level of care to patients with quick discharge and short-term follow-up. Effective use of ambulatory care has been shown to reduce hospital admissions by as much as 25% to 30% (Hamad & Connolly, 2018). Compared to patient care services performed in inpatient hospital settings, care provided by ambulatory centers for the same procedure is cost-effective due to the short-term nature of the stay. Hamad and Connolly (2018) posit that well-designed ambulatory care centers can meet the clinical and outpatient care needs of many hospital patients. The authors note that a well-designed ambulatory center includes having the necessary clinical staff and patient volume appropriate for providing optimum care. Additionally, it is important to identify patients who are at an acceptable risk level to receive care at an out-of-hospital facility; this is best determined by a senior clinician with the support of appropriate risk stratification tools.

Once the optimum patient population for a specific ambulatory care center is identified, the design of the center can be considered through the lens of inclusive design. While there has not been much research on inclusive design of nonacute care ambulatory settings, Zook et al. (2021) completed a case study of ambulatory care center layouts that included aspects of human factors design and universal design which builds toward a pathway of inclusive design and health equity.

The authors reviewed two very common yet divergent ambulatory center layouts and investigated the balance between achieving patient-centered care and support for healthcare providers. It was noted that patient-centered care is intensive and may lead to provider burnout (Zook et al., 2021). The two layouts included the onstage-offstage layout, where provider areas are discretely separate from patient access areas, and the center-stage layout, which links waiting areas and patient care areas and has highly visible corridors.

Relevant concepts in evaluating healthcare center layouts include opportunities for proximity of healthcare providers to each other, centrality of key work functions, intervisibility of patients, and opportunities for communication among healthcare team members. These concepts are greatly impacted by floor plan layouts; centralized provider stations and corridor layouts may determine how much or how little communication occurs among providers. An additional concern is visual and auditory privacy for both providers and patients. Zook et al. (2021) considered variables of communication, visibility, privacy, and proximity when evaluating best practices for ambulatory center layouts.

After review and investigation of two design layout types, center stage and on stage/off stage, it was determined that center-stage design layouts allowed for highest levels of patient-provider integration. The center-stage design layout creates greater potential for awareness and encounters of a variety of users such as nurses, doctors, and patients (Zook et al., 2021) (see Figure 10.1). The center-stage design generally

> centers on an "H"-shaped corridor space that both links the waiting area to the exam rooms and is continuous with the care team work area at the horizontal bar of the "H". This layout lets care staff see patients approach and monitor exam room doors from the teamwork area.
>
> (Zook et al., 2021, p. 228)

The center-stage floor plan impacts teamwork positively and allows for co-presence, communication, and intervisibility of multiple care team providers. This layout also requires less walking distance from provider to patient and allows for providers to have visibility of patients, hallways, and intake/waiting room areas. When considering human factors design and universal design, the study addressed several of the important factors, suggesting that the outcomes in the investigation are indicative of inclusive design. These factors include communication, user-friendly design, person-centered approach, simple and intuitive, perceptible information, and low physical effort (see Figure 10.2). These factors, while not all encompassing, can be essential in increasing inclusive access in patient care, thus broadening the opportunity for culturally sensitive care and health equity.

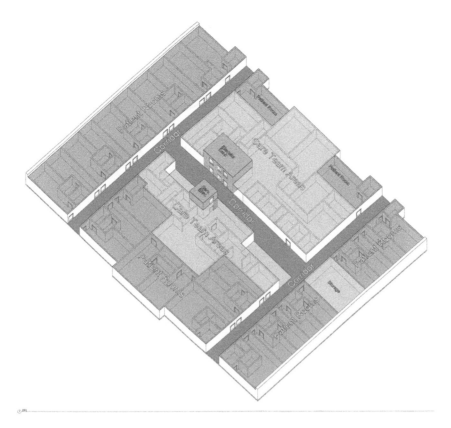

Figure 10.1 H corridor.

Emergency Medical Services

As was stated earlier in the chapter, health equity and inclusive design are relatively new areas of focus in research and practice, but this is especially true in emergency medical services (EMS). The National Association of Emergency Medical Services Physicians' (NAEMSP) Diversity, Equity, and Inclusion Committee published a position paper in February 2023 outlining the issues within EMS that require research and modification (Owusu-Ansah et al., 2023). The authors note that there are glaring disparities in patient outcomes when studying racial and ethnic minority populations and populations of women. These population groups do not receive time-sensitive care for acute coronary syndrome, out-of-hospital cardiac arrest, and stroke.

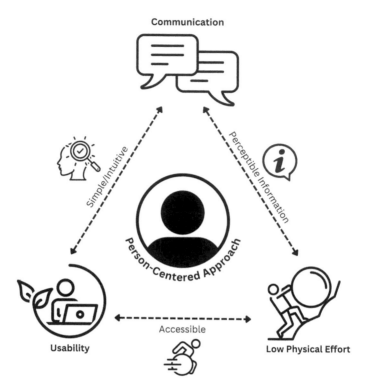

Figure 10.2 Person-centered approach.

Additionally, LGBTQ+ patients were rarely included in EMS research. Observable differences in healthcare outcomes are likely linked to provider implicit bias, social determinants of health, and healthcare access inequities. Some possible solutions to the health inequity include:

- Mentorship of EMS professionals from underrepresented backgrounds and expanding career pathways and opportunities to enhance diversity in the EMS workforce
- Development of programs that increase recruitment of women and minorities into the EMS workforce
- Providing cultural training and implicit bias training to all EMS professionals to prevent inequities in Black, Hispanic, Asian, and American Indian/Alaska Native patients from receiving less prehospital analgesia for pain

- Increasing patient education about life-threatening health conditions to prevent delay of care; it was found that Black, Asian, Hispanic, and female patients waited longer before seeking care for acute coronary syndrome (Owusu-Ansah et al., 2023)

Efforts to address glaring gaps in health equity have manifested emerging models that include a range of programs and treat-in-place protocol initiatives within EMS. These initiatives, which have gained significant traction since 2020, involve the dispatch of certified EMS professionals to patients' homes to assist with medication management, post-hospitalization patient care, assessment of mental health, and assessment of drug and alcohol use (Foubister et al., 2023). Often referred to as community paramedicine (CP) or mobile healthcare, these programs are important in developing pathways to health equity, inclusive access, and increased patient well-being. Community paramedicine programs (CPPs) have been developed and launched as a way of managing the approximately 27% of emergency room visits that could be prevented by appropriate use of primary care, ambulatory care, or proper medication management (Cistola et al., 2020). The CPPs receive referrals from primary care physicians, insurance providers, hospital staff, and/or home health agencies for patients who are likely to have a preventable hospital readmission within 30 days of discharge (Foubister et al., 2023).

The CPPs use the social determinants of health framework because they are common in rural environments and successfully address social factors that increase the likelihood of hospital readmission. They do so by making sure patients understand post-hospitalization care instructions, helping patients understand their existing or new diagnoses, ensuring patients have adequate environmental support within the home, connecting patients with primary care and follow-up appointments, determining which issues may impede a patient from self-management of their own health, assessing mental health, and assessing drug and alcohol use (Foubister et al., 2023). Cistola et al. (2020) conducted a study in Florida that paired 189 residents who had frequent emergency department use with CPs and resource coordinators.

The focus of the program is to address social determinants of health and resolve underlying issues of frequent ED utilization. Gainesville CRP [community resource paramedicine] personnel comprehensively evaluate and directly address social needs of patients including food security, transportation, employment, and disability access. Furthermore, Gainesville CRP personnel communicate with healthcare providers in real-time to ensure patients are adhering to their medication and treatment plans, convey details of their complete social picture, while also conducting detailed wellness checks on patients of particularly high-risk.

(Cistola et al., 2020, p. 4)

The researchers ultimately found that this approach led to a statistically significant reduction in future hospital admissions and emergency room visits. Similarly, Foubister et al. (2023) reported that CPPs reduced hospitalizations during the 30 days after intervention.

Overall, this care model can serve as a significant way to increase health equity and inclusive access to healthcare. Research has shown that patients recover faster when in safe, familiar, and comfortable environments (Rhode, 2021). Therefore, treating patients at home with the goal of preventing extended and repeated hospital stays has a positive impact on their recovery. This model is also cost-effective since estimates show that 4.4 billion dollars nationwide could be saved on preventable emergency department visits (Cistola et al., 2020). Hospitals and insurance companies have noted this cost-effective model and are increasingly funding CPPs, as the cost of the CP intervention is significantly less expensive than emergency room visits and hospitalizations. Additionally, EMS companies are interested in this concept as it reduces repeated calls to 911 and preventable hospital transports. Insurance companies are also beginning to reimburse EMS providers for CP services due to the cost-effective nature of this intervention (Foubister et al., 2023).

From an inclusive design perspective, CPPs address many of the concepts essential to development of inclusive healthcare access due to their treat-in-place design. What is yet to be studied is whether community paramedicine models require EMS providers to be well-versed in principles of diversity, equity, and inclusion to ensure inclusive access to each patient within their home environment. If this is achieved, it is seemingly a best practice for addressing health disparities that are caused by social determinants of health – one of the broader goals of inclusive healthcare design.

Human Factors Design for Ambulances

In 2015, the First Responders Group of the U.S. Department of Homeland Security developed the *Ambulance Patient Compartment Human Factors Design Guidebook* as a tool for EMS transportation systems (Avery et al., 2015). The guidebook is a thorough treatment of the subject of ambulance compartment safety and efficiency and covers human factors engineering, user-centered design, seating and restraints, equipment and supplies, storage, workspace, ingress and egress, communication, and ambulance types (Avery et al., 2015). The guide notes building spaces that are accessible and efficient for EMS professionals who are males in the 95th percentile as well as females who are in the 5th percentile; the guide also takes into consideration building safe spaces for children and the appropriate restraints needed. The guide provides instruction on safe lighting and building for effective communication among providers and between providers and patients. While extremely comprehensive, the guidebook focuses on EMS personnel performance and safety with few mentions of diverse populations and no mention of equity, patient-centered care, or inclusivity.

Design Considerations for Special Populations

Special populations of patients often require inclusion of specific design elements in healthcare spaces, yet these special design considerations can also be beneficial to the general population of patients. For the purpose of this chapter, we will focus on design for aging patients as well as pediatric patients with specific autism spectrum diagnoses, as these populations require numerous design supports which can inform design for all.

Aging Populations

Person-centered approaches to design for aging patients are important, as these patients often show decline during long-term hospital stays (Rhode, 2021). Personalized spaces include social and communal spaces that allow for social interactions with providers, visitors, and other patients. These communal spaces should be a place where patients can encounter providers and get their questions answered. Rhode emphasizes that "design for an aging population must include not only safeguards for health and welfare, but also opportunities for wellness, socializing, and thriving rather than declining" (2021). There are four areas of emphasis when designing for aging populations: lighting, acoustics, safe movement/mobility, and thermal environments; these elements offer safety as well as comfort (Rhode, 2021). Lighting is important, as visibility declines are common in older patients; placement of lighting and use of natural lighting can assist patients with reading signage and wayfinding through healthcare spaces. Acoustics are also relevant considering that declines in hearing are also common in aging populations. Important considerations for those who are hearing impaired include but are not limited to closed captioning on visual screens, volume of verbal conversations, volume of ambient music or other conversations in close proximity, and opportunities for auditory messages to be repeated. Safe movement is also a high priority, as falls in older patients can be challenging to overall health. Fall prevention and safe movement design considerations include the use of nonslip flooring materials, planning for smooth thresholds/transitions, handrails that can be easily accessed, and strategically placed seating along traveled pathways to allow for breaks. Lastly, the thermal environment is relevant, as older patients are often cold, while providers and staff are usually hot. Finding the right balance for ambient temperature with the capacity for personalizing preferred temperatures for older patients should be considered in the design process.

Overall, inclusive design for aging populations creates a pathway toward elimination of agism in healthcare spaces, an emphasis on safety as well as well-being, and a culture of respect. Piatkowski and Taylor (2016) emphasized, "There is an opportunity at hand for design to support the advancing needs of people as they age" and a way to "bridge the gap between basic human rights and higher human needs – for everyone" (p. 10). The aforementioned design supports include the majority of human factors design and universal design aspects that lead to inclusive design.

Autism Spectrum Disorders

The Centers for Disease Control and Prevention (2023) define autism spectrum disorders as a "developmental disability that can cause significant social, communication and behavioral challenges" (para. 1). Individuals on this spectrum often have sensory sensitivity that manifests as hyper- or hyposensitivity to sounds, smells, and visual stimuli (Peavey et al., 2020). These sensitivities can impact patients, especially pediatric patients, when they interact with healthcare systems. Peavy et al. (2020) posit five design guidelines that create an inclusive healthcare environment for individuals diagnosed with autism spectrum disorders, yet can benefit all patients.

The first guideline is predictability and intuitive navigation, which asks designers not to rely on use of signage for patient flows; instead, it urges designers to develop floor plan layouts that are intuitive and allow patients to view multiple areas and paths to where their next level of care is received. Predictability and intuitive navigation require the avoidance of blind corners where patients can be surprised by who or what is coming around the corner of the next hallway. Patients should be able to visually view reception areas, patient care areas, and their healthcare provider stations as they approach and leave.

The next guideline the authors described is prospect and refuge, which indicates that the healthcare environment mirrors a natural environment, where patients have choices of how little or how much interaction they prefer (Peavey et al., 2020). The authors point to the inclusion of spatial programs such as reading nooks in libraries and corner booths in restaurants, designed to allow patient views of larger, more crowded areas from a safe and enclosed distance. This suggests creating places where patients can feel safe yet fully aware of their surroundings.

The third guideline is personalization and choice, which recommends the development of spaces where patients can choose or curate their level of sensory stimulation. For example, patients should be allowed to select lighting intensity and color, sound volume and ambient sounds, and temperature. This guideline is also relevant to aging populations, as sensory levels are likely to have an impact on their safety and comfort levels.

The fourth guideline, sensory moderation and respite, creates opportunities within the design for patients to minimize sources of sensory inputs. This guideline requires that optimal patient flow be achieved to minimize areas of congestion and allows for areas of lower stimulation where patients cannot overhear loud conversations and can personalize and customize sensory inputs through the use of technology in design.

The last guideline shared by Peavy et al. (2020) is joy and engagement, which allows design to balance positive distraction with sensory overload. This guideline challenges designers to include areas that are comforting, interesting, and inviting to the patient; themes of nature or animals may be incorporated for younger patients. The authors share the following example from Our Lady of the Lake Children's Hospital in Baton Rouge, Louisiana.

At Our Lady of the Lake Children's Hospital in Baton Rouge, Louisiana, each department is themed according to one of the ecosystems found throughout the state using its own color palette, graphic feature walls representing the local flora, and "animal ambassadors." While neutrals comprise the bulk of the material palette, pops of color, and watercolor patterns highlight destinations like family lounges or nurse stations. On the unit, each patient room has a "front porch" following the color palette of the unit, nurse stations are outfitted with wall protection printed with watercolor imagery in matching colors, and PPE cabinets located between pairs of patient rooms feature nature-themed artwork (Peavy et al., 2020).

CASE STUDY

A 76-year-old male patient who was diagnosed with congestive heart failure (CHF) one year ago, high blood pressure five years ago, and has had diabetes for the last three months is being followed by his internal medicine doctor, as well as his cardiologist. He lives alone in a rural area and has his own vehicle, but rarely drives himself long distances. The patient has difficulty walking long distances, standing for longer than 10 to 20 minutes, maneuvering stairways and doorway thresholds, and dressing himself. He is normally compliant with his medications but at times he forgets to take his evening doses of medication.

While the patient's diabetes has been well-controlled for the past three months, two weeks ago he was discharged from his regional hospital after being admitted for complications related to CHF. He has a follow-up appointment with his physician in four days.

Today's presenting problem:

During a follow-up telephone call the patient reported that he was currently experiencing shortness of breath while lying in bed watching TV and he also noticed that his ankles were swollen. He says he thinks that he took his medications as directed for the past few days, but he can't really remember because he didn't write it down.

DISCUSSION QUESTIONS

1. Is this patient best treated in a hospital setting? Ambulatory care setting? Treat-in-place setting? Give a reason for your answer.
2. Name all relevant design considerations necessary for optimal treatment of the patient based on your response to question 1 (hospital, ambulatory care, treat-in-place).
3. Based on the patient's history and diagnoses, what inclusive design elements would be beneficial to him in a healthcare setting?
4. What social determinants of health might be relevant to the patient's current situation?

References

Ambulatory Surgery Center Association. (n.d.). *Quality of care in ambulatory surgery centers.* www.advancingsurgicalcare.com/advancingsurgicalcare/home

Avery, L., Jacobs, A., Moore, J., & Boone, C. (2015). *Ambulance patient compartment human factors design guidebook.* US Department of Homeland Security Science and Technology Directorate First Responders Group.

Centers for Disease Control and Prevention. (2022, December 8). *Social determinants of health at CDC.* Retrieved April 27, 2023, from www.cdc.gov/about/sdoh/index.html

Centers for Disease Control and Prevention. (2023, March 31). *Autism spectrum disorder.* Retrieved April 27, 2023, from www.cdc.gov/ncbddd/autism/index.html

Cistola, S. A., Bak, A. N., Guyer, L., Reed, L., Rooks, B., & Chacko, L. (2020). Approaches for improving health equity: The effect of the Gainesville community resource paramedic program on reducing emergency department utilization. *Research Square*, 1–15. https://doi.org/10.21203/rs.3.rs-87078/v1

Foubister, V., Hostetter, M., & Klein, S. (2023, March 24). Can community paramedicine improve health outcomes in rural America? The Commonwealth Fund. Retrieved April 27, 2023, from https://doi.org/10.26099/5zpy-rq24

Hamad, M. M. A. A., & Connolly, V. M. (2018). Ambulatory emergency care- improvement by design. *Clinical Medicine*, 18(1), 69–74. https//doi.org/10.7861/clinmedicine.18-1-69

Lanteigne, V. A., Rider, T. R., & Stratton, P. A. (n.d.). Advancing health equity through inclusive design. *Environments by Design: Health, Wellbeing and Place*, 78–89.

Owusu-Ansah, S., Tripp, R., Weisberg, S. N., Mercer, M. P., & Whitten-Chung, K. (2023). Essential principles to create an equitable, inclusive, and diverse EMS workforce and work environment: A position statement and resource document. *Prehospital Emergency Care*, 27(5), 552–556. https://doi.org/10.1080/10903127.2023.2187103

Peavey, E., Knox, R., & Reyers, E. (2020, April 28). Inclusive design for patients with autism spectrum disorders. *HCD Magazine*. Retrieved April 27, 2023, from https://healthcaredesignmagazine.com/trends/perspectives/inclusive-design-for-patients-with-autsm-spectrum-disorders/

Piatkowski, M., & Taylor, E. T. (2016). *Universal design: Designing for human needs (research brief)* (pp. 1–14). The Center for Health Design.

Rhode, J. (2021, December 29). *Designing healthcare spaces for an aging population.* Eypae. Retrieved April 27, 2023, from www.eypae.com/publication/2021/designing-healthcare-spaces-aging-population

Zook, J., Spence, T. J., & Joy, T. (2021). Balancing support for staff and patient centeredness through the design of immediate and relational space: A case study of ambulatory care center layouts. *Health Environments Research & Design Journal, 14*(1), 224–236. https//doi.org/10.1177/1937586720961554

11

PATIENT ROOM CONSIDERATIONS FOR DIFFERENT HEALTHCARE NEEDS AND SCALES

Keneshia Bryant-Moore

Introduction

In recent years, there has been a recognition of the need to develop inclusive healthcare settings that promote spaces that are safe, hospitable, and equitable. The goal of inclusive healthcare settings is to create a welcoming environment for all patients regardless of age, gender, race, ethnicity, religion, nationality, geographic region, socioeconomic status, disability, health insurance status, education level, health literacy, sexual orientation, gender identity, sex characteristics, mental health status, refugee or migrant background, and religion/spirituality (Marjadi et al., 2023).

In 2023, Marjadi et al. published *Twelve Tips for Inclusive Practice in Healthcare Setting*; the purpose of these practical tips are for healthcare administrators and providers to develop an inclusive healthcare practice and service delivery. It is particularly important for populations who are often overlooked in mainstream healthcare service delivery. To paraphrase, the tips include: 1) beware of assumptions and stereotypes; 2) replace labels with appropriate

DOI: 10.4324/9781003414902-13

terminology; 3) use inclusive language; 4) ensure inclusivity in the physical space; 5) use inclusive and appropriate signs and symbols; 6) ensure appropriate communication methods; 7) adopt a strength-based approach; 8) ensure inclusivity in healthcare research; 9) expand the scope of inclusive healthcare delivery; 10) advocate for a more inclusive healthcare system; 11) self-educate on diversity in all its forms; and 12) build individual and institutional commitments. These 12 tips for inclusive practice highlight the need to redefine what it means to be an inclusive healthcare organization by incorporating facility design in healthcare delivery spaces (Marjadi et al., 2023).

But additional considerations are needed for equitable and inclusive healthcare facilities. The author presents information about some principles of healthcare environments and how they can be incorporated; specifics regarding the built environment are discussed, and the discussion ends with considerations for patient rooms at various scales and settings.

Five Principles of Creating Healthcare Environments

Five general principles should be considered when planning and designing equitable, inclusive healthcare settings that promote safe care for patients. The five principles are 1) patient-centeredness, 2) patient engagement, 3) responsiveness, 4) continuous refinement, 5) value and respect.

Principle 1: Patient-Centeredness

Patient-centeredness integrates patients, values, preferences, and goals into clinical care. Achieving patient-centered care and positive, constructive communication in provider-patient clinical interactions is complex and can be impacted by institutional structures, personal/behavioral-related barriers, and the environment. Patient-centered care comprises several components that affect the way health systems deliver care to patients, including how both the systems and facilities are designed and managed. Patient-centered care is engaging, collaborative, coordinated, and accessible. It considers and incorporates the patient's surroundings, environment, amenities, and physical comfort and the needs of their family, friends, and caregivers in healthcare delivery. Patients, their caregivers, and their families are also expected to be members of the care team, participating in decision-making at the patient and system level. Because the presence of caregivers and family members in the care setting is encouraged and facilitated in the patient-centered care model, accommodation with the care delivery setting must also incorporate their needs as well. This can be a benefit for patients and healthcare organizations, as evidence suggests that patient-centeredness leads to improved satisfaction ratings among patients and their caregivers and families (New England Journal of Medicine [NEJM] Catalyst, 2017).

Principle 2: Patient Engagement

Historically, patient engagement has focused on building patient autonomy and self-determination, with the goals of promoting patient confidence and trust in the clinician-patient relationship, improving knowledge, and setting reasonable expectations (Krist et al., 2017). Patient engagement is also essential for promoting a positive patient experience and satisfaction. Strategies for patient engagement at a healthcare system level include engaging patients and families in 1) serving on advisory boards or councils, 2) attending health administration meetings, 3) participating on project teams, 4) presenting at forums/workshops, 5) providing instruction for healthcare professionals in training, and 6) providing consultation (Bennett et al., 2020).

Principle 3: Responsiveness

Responsiveness is how well the health system meets the reasonable expectations of patients, caregivers, and families for the non-health-enhancing aspects of the health system. Darby et al., (2003), in collaboration with the World Health Organization (WHO), issued their strategy for measuring responsiveness. Responsiveness embraces aspects of respect of human rights and includes seven elements: dignity (the state or quality of being worthy of honor or respect), confidentiality (privacy), autonomy (independence), prompt attention (engaging the patient to determine action), social support (having people to turn to in times of need or crisis), basic amenities (essential things to make life easier), and choice of provider (selected as the patient's best healthcare provider) (Darby et al., 2003; Robone et al., 2011). These elements provide guidance for healthcare organizations on how to respond to the needs of patients, caregivers, and families.

Principle 4: Continuous Refinement

Continuous refinement is the process of planning and implementing ongoing improvement strategies and practices within and to the healthcare facility. The primary goal of these strategies is to improve patient experiences, prioritizing satisfaction, safety, sense of belonging, and being "seen." Continuous refinement can be combined with quality improvement when considering the entire healthcare delivery system, and includes actions taken to improve the healthcare service. To establish this process as an integrated aspect of the healthcare system, it is necessary to monitor and consistently evaluate improvement efforts and outcomes (McCalman et al., 2018).

Principle 5: Value and Respect

The value and respect principle is approached broadly and it includes addressing the diversity of patients, the delivery of quality healthcare services, and the design of inclusive healthcare settings. The principle requires that patients be treated with dignity, courtesy, care, and compassion. Healthcare disparities and inequities are notable among members of underserved communities, such as African American/Black, Latino, Indigenous and Native American, Asian Americans, Pacific Islanders, and other persons of color; members of religious minorities; lesbian, gay, bisexual, transgender, and queer (LGBTQ+) persons; persons with disabilities; rural residents; and persons otherwise adversely affected by persistent poverty or inequality (Agency for Healthcare Research and Quality, 2021). Special consideration is needed for these populations who have experienced historic marginalization and discrimination in all aspects of society, including healthcare settings. Ensuring that these patients know that they are valued and respected can overcome issues of patients from these populations feeling excluded, mistrusting healthcare services, and/or being hesitant about accessing services. Table 11.1 depicts the principles that should be considered by healthcare environments.

Incorporating the Five Principles of Creating Healthcare Environments

The design and creation of inclusive healthcare facilities is essential for patients from diverse backgrounds to feel included. Inclusion in healthcare

Table 11.1 Five Principles of Creating Healthcare Environments

Patient-centeredness	The integration of a patient's values, preferences, and goals into their clinical care
Patient engagement	The active involvement of patients (and caregivers) in their own care
Responsiveness	How the health system meets the reasonable expectations of patients, caregivers, and family
Continuous refinement	The process of planning and implementing ongoing improvement strategies and practices
Value and respect	Treating patients with dignity, courtesy, care, and compassion

refers to the intentional, ongoing effort to ensure that diverse people with different identities can fully participate in all aspects of the healthcare organization (Tan, 2019). This means that the patient's, caregiver's, and family's preferences, values, cultural traditions, and socioeconomic conditions are respected. In an effort to prioritize the patient experience and to meet the needs of a full range of diverse patients, healthcare environments are required to address patients' various physical, sensory, and cognitive needs (Myerson & West, 2015). Healthcare organizations should strive to provide an environment that is welcoming and safe and provides a sense of belonging. Therefore, it is important to know and understand the patient population and community being served in any given healthcare setting, considering patient satisfaction and positive experience according to unique identity. Other data is also required to obtain a complete understanding of the patient population and their needs. It is important to note the patient population, which could be based on the geographical region served, insurance carriers accepted, types of services offered, and/or other factors.

Connections to the Built Environment

Regarding the patient experience, many discount the connection between patient rooms and other parts of the built environment. The built environment is defined as the physical makeup of where we live, learn, work, pray, and play (Young et al., 2020). This includes homes, businesses, streets and sidewalks, public spaces, transportation options, public art, and other features in the environment that are made by humans. The buildings and facilities that make up healthcare systems are included in this broader definition of built environment, and patient rooms are a subset of healthcare systems. The built environment as it relates to patient rooms can have a profound impact on patient care, support, and safety. The goal of every organization should be to maintain safe, aesthetically pleasing, high-quality, well-designed spaces that promote connectivity to other features on healthcare campuses and the built environment as a whole. Beautiful buildings and surroundings not only promote pride in the neighborhood but can also have a positive impact on the morale and overall well-being of patients, visitors, and employees. Thus, patient rooms should not be thought of as singular, static spaces during the design process, but as a part of a singular experience beginning when patrons arrive at the facility.

Several features can be incorporated into the design of healthcare facilities to enhance the patient experience. Gardens, water features, outdoor sitting areas, scenic walkways, and other special characteristics can be incorporated into the design of these facilities. Though many in-patient facilities already have one or more of these features, they are often not included in the design of smaller facilities or those that primarily provide outpatient care services and are not a part of the journey that patrons take as they enter the site and travel up to patient rooms. Patients, caregivers, and visitors spend several hours per week in outpatient healthcare facilities for treatments such as chemotherapy and dialysis. Their surroundings can have a significant impact on their mental state and well-being. Therefore, incorporating these considerations in these areas can be beneficial.

Healthcare Facility Exterior

The physical exteriors of a healthcare facility should be welcoming, providing a lasting first impression among patients, caregivers, and families of being valued and appreciated. In addition to the considerations described in the built environment section, there are other strategies that could contribute to an inclusive healthcare facility exterior space: 1) Signage – The name of the facility, parking, and entrances should be in visible, well-lit areas, with the use of appropriate vocabulary written in the languages of the populations served. 2) Parking – Vehicle parking areas should be easily identified, and there should be an appropriate number of accessible parking spaces available, including unloading zones for wheelchair, van, or chair lifts to either side. Unloading zones and parking for other modes of transportation, like medical transportation, buses, and vehicles, should be provided, depending on the location of the healthcare facility and the types of care they provide. Bike racks should be provided for those who choose to ride their bicycle to the facility. 3) Transit – Bus stops and nearby waiting stations for other modes of transit, such as light rail systems, should be accessible and covered or partially enclosed to protect patrons from adverse weather conditions. 4) Exterior walkways – Sidewalks and pathways facilities should be clearly identifiable, clear of obstructions, and accessible for all users. These considerations play an important part in the connectivity between the larger built environment and patient rooms.

Healthcare Facility Interior

Healthcare facility interiors are the first spatial contact between patrons and healthcare facilities. Before patrons get access to patient rooms, they must pass through a series of spaces serving a variety of patient needs and may be required to engage with the healthcare facility staff. One such space is the waiting room, where the use of *patient-directed technology* has increased over the years and includes features like kiosks for check-in/registration, tablets for patient-reported data collection, and smart screens for health education. Waiting room tablets have also been used for patients with complex health issues as a way to identify and set discussion topic priorities for their healthcare visit (Lyles et al., 2016). A patient education space with computers for patients and visitors to use is ideal for those who may not have access at home (Horwitz-Bennet, 2014).

The design of waiting areas can help prevent disease transmission and reduce the spread of contagious illnesses. Since the beginning of the COVID-19 pandemic in 2020, waiting rooms have been identified as areas with a high risk of spreading disease. In pediatric facilities, children often touch and play in close proximity with other children who they do not know in waiting rooms, increasing the risk of direct infection. Shared toys and books should be regularly disinfected after use to prevent spread of disease. Additionally, inclusive play spaces should address all sensory needs and levels of pediatric patients, as well as therapeutic seating options from swings to rocking chairs (Shaw, 2019).

Another space is the restrooms. When creating a space of inclusivity, the restroom options and needs available to patients and their visitors within the facility should be taken into consideration. Three areas of interest include meeting the needs of patients with disabilities/mobility issues, gender-inclusive and family restrooms, and quality of the restroom. Patrons with disabilities and mobility issues should have access to handicap-accessible restrooms. Americans with Disabilities Act (ADA) standards for restrooms impact the direction of toilet stall door swings; stall sizes; handle heights; and the height of the toilet, sink/vanity, counter, soap and paper towel dispensers, hand dryers, and the mounting locations of handrails. Other considerations like lever-style door handles and nonslip flooring could improve the accessibility and safety of restrooms.

The cleanliness of the restroom should be a priority. The availability of feminine hygiene products and trash bins to easily discard used products is important. Trash bins should be available near the sinks and entry/exit doors, and toilet seat covers should be available in each stall. Restrooms should also be well lit and can even incorporate the use of UV-C disinfection lighting for water, air, and surfaces. In an effort to keep the environment fresh, the use of automatic air fresheners that spray perfumes at regular intervals may be used. For those who desire to make the restroom an even more pleasant experience, music can also be played.

Traditionally, healthcare facilities that serve a large number of people at a time, like hospitals, have offered gang-style gendered restrooms with multiple toilet stalls, along with single-occupancy restrooms for individuals or families. Smaller facilities like outpatient clinics will have single-occupancy restrooms, usually one each for men and women. Recent years have seen the introduction of all-gender restrooms. All-gender restrooms, also referred to as gender-neutral restrooms, unisex restrooms, and gender-inclusive restrooms, are facilities that anyone can use, rejecting the notion of gender as a binary. The advocacy for all-gender restrooms has largely been promoted to benefit transgender, nonbinary, and non-gender-conforming persons, but others, including people those with body image issues, those who require the assistance of a caregiver of a different gender, and parents with small children of a different gender, also benefit from these types of facilities. There are potential drawbacks to all-gender restrooms such as discomfort of some patrons to share the space with others of different genders. This discomfort may lead to conflict, causing some to avoid the use of restroom facilities due to feelings of awkwardness or lack of privacy. Although this could be costly, providing a variety of restroom types could ensure that everyone feels accepted and included. Regardless of the type of restroom offered, restrooms should be labeled clearly with text and images so patients and visitors can understand what features are provided.

Patient Rooms in Inpatient Healthcare Facilities

Patients, families, and visitors will immediately notice the ambience and aesthetics of the healthcare facility interior. This includes lighting – both natural and artificial – art, décor, scents, colors, furnishings, fixtures, climate, and other aspects. Patients also observe signs and clues of diversity and openness to diverse groups and identities. Signs and symbols within healthcare facilities send messages; therefore, designers and administrators should be intentional about the kinds of messages being communicated to patients and visitors and how they are interpreting them.

Design and Décor

The design and décor of the patient room should combine function, safety, and comfort. If properly designed, they support a significant role in healing, wellness, and calming the anxiety of patients, their families, and visitors. Furniture should be comfortable and designed for a variety of diverse body types and abilities. Furniture should also be safe, durable, easy to clean, and considering the lessons from the COVID-19 pandemic, have the ability to be arranged as needed for social distancing, grouping, and to prevent the spread of disease. Signage and symbols posted within patient rooms can promote inclusion and belonging. For example, the display of a pride flag outside patient rooms signifies solidarity for the LGBTQ+ population. These symbols can serve as an indication of safety and belonging for patients who often face bias in healthcare settings.

Confidentiality and Privacy

The designers of patient rooms should also consider the confidentiality and privacy of patients and their families. Risks to breaches in confidentiality may occur if patients, families, and visitors overhear private conversations between healthcare providers and/or staff and other patients, families, and visitors. Patient confidence and trust can be broken if breaches in confidentiality occur.

Patient Room Bathrooms

There are specific considerations for patient bathrooms in inpatient healthcare facilities, usually found ensuite, that expand upon the previous discussion about healthcare facility restrooms. Patient bathrooms, often called *dedicated clinical toilet rooms*, fall into one of two categories in terms of inpatient healthcare facilities. The first category speaks to specific needs in *medical or surgical patient rooms*. Similar to bathrooms in hospitality suites, these bathrooms boast hotel-like finishes and fixtures that have the durability of hospital-grade equipment (Costello, 2021). Easy-to-clean finishes like fiberglass-reinforced plastic (FRP), nonslip flooring to minimize falls, intravenous (IV) hooks, and accessible features like grab bars are all present in *dedicated clinical toilet rooms* (Costello, 2021).

The second category is *intensive care units*, which are usually present in rooms where the patients have limited mobility or consciousness or have health conditions that require assistance from healthcare professionals. In this case, patient bathrooms have the same features as *medical or surgical patient rooms*, but with additional features that allow for a shift in their function (Costello, 2021). These features include assistive technologies such as call buttons and phones, roll-in showers, and accessible tilt mirrors. Some hospitals have made the shift to bathrooms that act as soiled utility spaces and contain features like flush sinks for washing bedpans and hand-washing sinks; however, these types of bathroom facilities are not ideal for visiting family members (Costello, 2021).

To ensure that patient rooms are safe spaces that promote healing, dedicated clinical toilet rooms should be located at the interior head wall, allowing for clear window sightlines for exterior views and natural light. Patient rooms should allow for clear pathways to ensure safe travel between patient beds and ensuite patient bathrooms (Horwitz-Bennet, 2014). Some design firms suggest *dedicated clinical toilet room* doors either be sliding or double doors to ensure an accessible opening that is at least four feet wide. All dedicated clinical toilet rooms are designed to ADA standards, with grab bars installed at appropriate locations, enough space for at least a five-foot turning radius, sinks at an accessible height, and smooth flooring to avoid obstructions that may cause falls (U.S. Department of Justice, 2010). These measures support the care of patients occupying patient rooms for extended periods of time, providing an inclusive experience for them and their families.

Patient Examination Rooms in Outpatient Settings

When designing patient examination rooms in outpatient settings, additional factors require consideration regarding inclusivity and patient experience. The focus on the design and décor of the patient examination room will be on two areas: patient-provider communication and technology.

The use of technological devices (e.g., desktop computers, tablets) for patient charting often requires healthcare providers to complete data entry during appointment visits. Research suggests that the examination room design and layout can impact provider-patient communication and interaction, in addition to patient comfort and privacy. For example, positioning furniture and equipment so that the provider always faces the patient supports eye contact and improves communication. Additionally, patient access to the computer screen has shown to increase provider information sharing and more time engaging patients in conversation about the information on the screen (Ajiboye et al., 2015). The distance and orientation between chairs, the examination table, privacy curtain, and door are important for protecting patient and family comfort and privacy (Zamani & Harper, 2019).

Patient examination rooms in recent years are being utilized as consultation rooms for specialty providers via telemedicine (Burke et al., 2023). The term "telemedicine" describes information and communication technologies that support the delivery of healthcare services from a geographical distance (Sood et al., 2007). Depending on the type of specialty service being provided, there may or may not be a healthcare provider in the room with the patient during all aspects of the care delivery and interaction. Therefore, consideration of the patients' needs and how they may impact the design of the room is paramount.

Innovation in Nontraditional Healthcare Settings

Nontraditional healthcare spaces for telemedicine in community settings, such as schools, places of worship, and places employment, can provide opportunities for a more inclusive approach to care delivery (Edgerton, 2017; Kodjebacheva et al., 2023). Healthcare administrators can collaborate with these community institutions to ensure the environment promotes equity, inclusion, and diversity for patients.

The use of technology is often considered a step in the right direction toward improving the health and well-being of patients. By increasing access, organizing patient records more efficiently, providing access to health management tools, and providing patient access to health information, health outcomes can be improved significantly (NORC at the University of Chicago, 2013). Unfortunately, not all patients have access to the technology services required for the administrations of telemedicine. For example, during the COVID-19 pandemic there was an overwhelming increase in the use of telemedicine for patient appointments; many patients in rural settings, however, had limited access to broadband internet or suffered from signal inadequacies in their area. Additionally, patients with low digital literacy, those who had not used technology, or those who do not have access to computers or smartphones were left with the inability to access adequate telehealth services.

Conclusion

The aim of inclusive healthcare settings to create a welcoming environment for all patients can be achieved. The application of the five guiding principles of equitable, inclusive healthcare settings can assist in that achievement. The collaborative design of healthcare facilities will have an impact on patient safety, satisfaction, and health outcomes and will likely have a positive impact on providers, staff, visitors, and administrators.

KEY POINTS

- Five general principles of equitable, inclusive healthcare settings: patient-centeredness, patient engagement, responsiveness, continuous refinement, value, and respect.
- Design of the exterior and interior features of the healthcare facility impact patient safety, experience, and health outcomes.
- Future trends include healthcare facilities partnering with community dwelling organizations for telemedicine delivery. These settings require diligence in providing equitable, inclusive spaces.

ACTIVITY

Go to a local clinic, hospital, or other healthcare delivery setting and conduct an equitable and inclusive visual survey of the facility. Use the information in the chapter to guide your assessment. Visualize the facility from a patient perspective, taking note of the positive and negative aspects of the built environment and the healthcare facility. Also, consider what questions you would ask the healthcare administrators about the facility.

References

Agency for Healthcare Research and Quality. (2021, June). *About priority populations.* Retrieved July 22, 2023, from www.ahrq.gov/priority-populations/about/index.html

Ajiboye, F., Dong, F., Moore, J., Kallail, K. J., & Baughman, A. (2015). Effects of revised consultation room design on patient-physician communication. HERD, 8(2), 8–17. https://doi.org/10.1177/1937586714565604

Bennett, W., Pitts, S., Aboumatar, H., Sharma, R., Smith, B. M., Das, A., Day, J., Holzhauer, K., & Bass, E. B. (2020, August). *Strategies for patient, family, and caregiver engagement* (Technical Brief, No. 36). Agency for Healthcare Research and Quality (US) Evidence Summary. Retrieved July 22, 2023, from www.ncbi.nlm.nih.gov/books/NBK561683/

Burke, G. V., Osman, K. A., Lew, S. Q., Ehrhardt, N., Robie, A. C., Amdur, R. L., Martin, L. W., & Sikka, N. (2023). Improving specialty care access via telemedicine. *Telemedicine Journal and E-Health: The Official Journal of the American Telemedicine Association*, 29(1), 109–115. https://doi.org/10.1089/tmj.2021.0597

Costello, J. (2021, March 24). *Re-thinking the design of healthcare restrooms: Margulies Peruzzi – design for the way you work.* Retrieved August 7, 2023, from https://mparchitectsboston.com/re-thinking-the-design-of-healthcare-restrooms/

Darby, C., Valentine, N., DeSilva, A., Murray, C. J., & World Organization. (2003). *World Health Organization (WHO): Strategy on measuring responsiveness.* Retrieved July 22, 2023, from https://apps.who.int/iris/handle/10665/68703

Edgerton, S. S. (2017, Fall). A pilot study investigating employee utilization of corporate telehealth services. *Perspectives in Health Information Management*, 14.

Horwitz-Bennet, B. (Ed.). (2014, June 25). Patient bathroom designs balance style and safety. *Healthcare Design Magazine.*

Kodjebacheva, G. D., Tang, C., Groesbeck, F., Walker, L., Woodworth, J., & Schindler-Ruwisch, J. (2023). Telehealth use in pediatric care during the COVID-19 pandemic: A qualitative study on the perspectives of caregivers. *Children (Basel, Switzerland)*, 10(2), 311. https://doi.org/10.3390/children10020311

Krist, A. H., Tong, S. T., Aycock, R. A., & Longo, D. R. (2017). Engaging patients in decision-making and behavior change to promote prevention. *Studies in Health Technology and Informatics*, 240, 284–302.

Lyles, C., Altschuler, A., Chawla, N., Kowalski, C., McQuillan, D., Bayliss, E., Heisler, M., & Grant, R. (2016). User-centered design of a tablet waiting room tool for complex patients to prioritize discussion topics for primary care visits. *JMIR Mhealth Uhealth*, 4(3), e108. Retrieved May 14, 2023, from https://mhealth.jmir.org/2016/3/e108; https//doi.org/10.2196/mhealth.6187

Marjadi, B., Flavel, J., Baker, K., Glenister, K., Morns, M., Triantafyllou, M., Strauss, P., Wolff, B., Procter, A. M., Mengesha, Z., Walsberger, S., Qiao, X., & Gardiner, P. A. (2023). Twelve tips for inclusive practice in healthcare settings. *International Journal of Environmental Research and Public Health*, 20(5), 4657. https://doi.org/10.3390/ijerph20054657

McCalman, J., Bailie, R., Bainbridge, R., McPhail-Bell, K., Percival, N., Askew, D., Fagan, R., & Tsey, K. (2018). Continuous quality improvement and comprehensive primary health care: A systems framework to improve service quality and health outcomes. *Frontiers in Public Health*, 6, 76. https://doi.org/10.3389/fpubh.2018.00076

Myerson, J., & West, J. (2015, November 12–13). *Make it better: How universal design principles can have an impact on healthcare services to improve the patient experience.* Universal Design in Education.

New England Journal of Medicine (NEJM) Catalyst. (2017). *What is patient-centered care?* Retrieved April 29, 2023, from https://catalyst.nejm.org/doi/full/10.1056/CAT.17.0559

NORC at the University of Chicago. (2013, May). *Revised briefing paper: Understanding the impact of health IT in underserved communities and those with health disparities.* Prepared for the U.S. Department of Health and Human Services. Retrieved May 1, 2023, from www.healthit.gov/sites/default/files/pdf/hit-underserved-communities-health-disparities.pdf

Robone, S., Rice, N., & Smith, P. C. (2011). Health systems' responsiveness and its characteristics: A cross-country comparative analysis. *Health Services Research*, 46(6pt. 2), 2079–2100. https://doi.org/10.1111/j.1475-6773.2011.01291.x

Shaw, D. (2019). The hidden risks of the waiting room: Confidentiality and cross-infection. *The British Journal of General Practice: The Journal of the Royal College of General Practitioners*, 69(683), 299. https://doi.org/10.3399/bjgp19X703925

Sood, S., Mbarika, V., Jugoo, S., Dookhy, R., Doarn, C., Prakash, N., & Merrell, R. (2007). What is telemedicine? A collection of 104 peer-reviewed perspectives and theoretical underpinnings. *Telemedicine and E-Health*, 13, 573–590. https//doi.org/10.1089/tmj.2006.0073

Tan, T. (2019). Principles of inclusion, diversity, access, and equity. *The Journal of Infectious Diseases*, 220(15), S30–S32. https://doi.org/10.1093/infdis/jiz198

U.S. Department of Justice. (2010). *2010 ADA standards for accessible design.* https://archive.ada.gov/regs2010/2010ADAStandards/2010ADAstandards.htm#medicalfacilities

Young, D., Cradock, A., Eyler, A., Fenton, M., Pedroso, M., Sallis, J., & Whitsel, L. (2020). Creating built environments that expand active transportation and active living across the United States: A policy statement from the American heart association. *Circulation*, 142(11), e167–e183.

Zamani, Z., & Harper, E. (2019). Exploring the effects of clinical exam room design on communication, technology interaction, and satisfaction. *HERD: Health Environments Research & Design Journal*, 12(4), 99–115. https//doi.org/10.1177/1937586719826055

CHAPTER 11 EXAMPLE: PATIENT ENGAGEMENT METHOD

KENESHIA BRYANT-MOORE

"Patient engagement is defined as the desire and capability to actively choose to participate in care in a way uniquely appropriate to the individual, in cooperation with a healthcare provider or institution, for the purposes of maximizing outcomes or improving experiences of care" (Higgins et al., 2017, p. 30). It is valuable to not only understand the perspectives of patients but also to take action and make meaningful changes to the built environment. A research study conducted in Charleston, South Carolina (Newman et al., 2009) used photovoice in a participatory action research project to identify the needs of persons with disabilities and then make a change. Photovoice is a qualitative "participatory method that has community participants use photography, and stories about their photographs, to identify and represent issues of importance to them" (Nykiforuk et al., 2011, p. 103). The photovoice method engages and empowers patients and caregivers to share and describe their viewpoint as opposed to relying on healthcare providers and administrators to make assumptions. The photographs provide visual evidence to help identify and address issues of accessibility in the community.

In healthcare facility design, photovoice enables patients to record their thoughts and beliefs about the existing facility, including the strengths and concerns. This visual aid with descriptions can be a powerful resource for those planning to develop or renovate existing patient care areas in the facility. The information gained can also be used to promote dialogue between healthcare administrators, patients, and the community they serve.

References

Higgins, T., Larson, E., & Schnall, R. (2017). Unraveling the meaning of patient engagement: A concept analysis. *Patient Education and Counseling*, 100(1), 30–36. https://doi.org/10.1016/j.pec.2016.09.002

Newman, S., Maurer, D., Jackson, A., Saxon, M., Jones, R., & Reese, G. (2009). Gathering the evidence: Photovoice as a tool for disability advocacy. *Progress in Community Health Partnerships: Research, Education, and Action*, 3(2), 139–144. https://doi.org/10.1353/cpr.0.0074

Nykiforuk, C. I., Vallianatos, H., & Nieuwendyk, L. M. (2011). Photovoice as a method for revealing community perceptions of the built and social environment. International Journal of Qualitative Methods, 10(2), 103–124. https://doi.org/10.1177/160940691101000201

12

THE DESIGN OF RESIDENTIAL SPACES FOR HEALTHCARE

Kiwana T. McClung

Introduction

The need for in-home healthcare has become more pronounced over the last few years as transportation challenges, healthcare facility capacity, and the challenges of the COVID-19 pandemic have made it difficult to comprehensively address the healthcare needs of our population. The Centers for Disease Control and Prevention (CDC) reports that there are a little over 650,000 inpatient beds in the United States in 2023 and over 70% of those beds are currently occupied. With the U.S. population over 335 million, and even more numbers in other countries, one can understand why the need for in-home health care is so pressing (U.S. Census Bureau). There are other realities that support the case for in-home health care provisions. According to the U.S. Census Bureau, the decade between 2010 and 2020 saw both the largest and fastest growth in the elderly population since the nineteenth century. For the first time since 1880, the population over 65 years of age comprised more than 16% of the total U.S. population. This sharp rise can be attributed to the Baby Boomers, a generation of individuals born after

DOI: 10.4324/9781003414902-14

World War II between 1946 and 1964 (Caplan & Rabe, 2023). With the last of the Baby Boomers turning 65 right before 2030, it is clear that additional considerations and provisions will need to be made for caring for such a large population of elderly citizens.

One of these considerations is the current housing crisis. The National Low Income Housing Coalition estimates that the United States is currently facing a shortage of over 7 million affordable, available rental homes (National Low Income Housing Coalition [NLIHC], 2023). This figure becomes even more stark when one considers the need for affordable housing that supports those with mobile disabilities. Currently, all federally assisted new-construction residential housing developments containing five or more units must ensure that 12% of the units, or at least one unit, adheres to the requirements of the Americans with Disabilities (ADA) Act, with an additional 2% slated for those with visual and auditory disabilities (HUD-DOJ, 2008). While these provisions and standards are great, they do not come close to meeting the current need for accessible housing that supports individuals throughout their lives (U.S. Access Board, 1984). One way to address this shortage is by embracing design and construction strategies that allow individuals to age in place, lessening the need for elders to leave or sell their homes due to the lack of accessibility features (Steinfeld & Maisel, 2012). The additions and renovations that would need to take place to facilitate the continuous presence of individuals as they age are also necessary for those who receive in-home health care.

The concept of in-home health care is not a new one, but it has shifted over the years, becoming more frequent, specialized, and targeted. Now, considering the rising number of elderly and the healthcare needs they will undoubtedly have, the concept is perhaps more relevant than ever (Caplan & Rabe, 2023). This concept and its need were starkly demonstrated during the COVID-19 pandemic, when having in-home health care services was the safer option to traveling to a healthcare facility and possibly contracting the virus. Home health care services allow for both convenience and more holistic understanding for healthcare professionals of the obstacles patients must navigate during activities of daily living (ADL). This system allows various healthcare practitioners to provide quality care to patients through home visits, in a manner that is patient-centered and cost-effective (Song et al., 2021). However, it is important to ensure that accessibility and universal design strategies are considered.

Accessibility and Strategies for Universal Design

One of the largest concerns when addressing in-home health care is the need for accessible and universal design strategies. Accessibility concerns the facilitation of access to spaces and structures (U.S. Access Board, 1984). These standards govern considerations such as access, clearances, routes of travel, adaptability, accessibility elements such as grab bars, refuge spaces, and even assistive features. These features facilitate access and the ability for an individual to remain in the home throughout their lifespan. It is important to note that accessibility standards are not holistic in cultivating access, only requiring a minimum required for access.

Additionally, though we now have federal laws mandating the inclusion of accessible design features, the static nature of existing structures built prior to the passing of the ADA in 1968 make it difficult to achieve true accessibility, and what is achieved is often stigmatizing. Accessibility measures that require users to utilize back door or service entrances force those with disabilities to take circuitous routes, deny users experiences, compromise their safety, or rob users of their dignity; they fulfill ADA requirements but do more harm than good to the people affected (Steinfeld & Maisel, 2012). Universal design, however, is much more comprehensive, yet much less prescriptive.

Universal design is the design and cultivation of products and built environments that promote access, understanding, and usability to the greatest extent possible for all human beings regardless of ability, age, or size, without the need for adaptation or specialized design (Steinfeld & Maisel, 2012; Center for Universal Design, 1997). Universal design emerged from the disability rights movement and focuses on removing unnecessary barriers to access and improving the usability of built and virtual environments (Steinfeld & Maisel, 2012). Universal design as a philosophy is broad, containing aspects of accessibility, ergonomics, functionality, and sociospatial considerations. It is also an evolutionary process that hinges upon continuous improvement, is dependent on the resources available, and is considerate of the context that one is designing for. The core principle of universal design is that it is human-centered, placing the needs of people above profit, tradition, and commercial interests. Steinfeld and Maisel (2012) created a new definition for universal design that seems much more appropriate when considering the creation of inclusive and accessible healthcare spaces:

"Universal design is a process that enables and empowers a diverse population by improving human performance, health and wellness, and social participation" (p. 29).

The Center for Universal Design promotes seven principles, established by a working group led by the late Ronald Mace, an architect and disability advocate at North Carolina State University's School of Design (Center for Universal Design, 1997). The principles, listed in Table 12.1, serve as a litmus test for inclusive spaces, both physical and virtual; the more principles a space adheres to, the more inclusive it is. Design for healthcare is considered a related field to universal design, with both realms of design consideration employing evidence-based design. The creation of products and healthcare spaces that reduce the transmission of infectious diseases protects the well-being of healthcare providers and considers the various language barriers that may arise in healthcare interactions; this requires a universal design approach that centers both patient and caregiver well-being.

Design Strategies for Aging in Place

There can only be a need for in-home health care if individuals have to return home for a period of recovery or remain in their home throughout the course of their life. In the beginning of this chapter, the elderly were identified as a group with the greatest need in this regard due to the shifting demographics of elderly individuals, the increased likelihood of frailty that comes with age, and the advancements in healthcare that are allowing people to live longer, healthier lives (Caplan & Rabe, 2023). The existing stock of age-restricted housing that can accommodate the needs of elderly individuals is not enough to support the entirety of the elderly population we currently have, much less the increasing numbers of elderly we will have to accommodate over the next decades (Steinfeld & Maisel, 2012). This reality necessitates that as many elderly individuals as possible are able to remain in their homes throughout the duration of their lives, negating the need to build additional housing/healthcare facilities to accommodate the demand. If people are to remain in their homes while aging, residential spaces and structures need to be adapted and renovated to accommodate people with a much wider range of health conditions, abilities, needs, and equipment than traditional residential homes allow for. Universal design should assuredly

Table 12.1 The Seven Principles of Universal Design

Principles	Guidelines
Principle 1: Equitable Use The design is useful and marketable to people with diverse abilities.	1a. Provide the same means of use for all users: identical whenever possible; equivalent when not. 1b. Avoid segregating or stigmatizing any users. 1c. Provisions for privacy, security, and safety should be equally available to all users. 1d. Make the design appealing to all users.
Principle 2: Flexibility in Use The design accommodates a wide range of individual preferences and abilities.	2a. Provide choice in methods of use. 2b. Accommodate right- or left-handed access and use. 2c. Facilitate the user's accuracy and precision. 2d. Provide adaptability to the user's pace.
Principle 3: Simple and Intuitive Use Use of the design is easy to understand, regardless of the user's experience, knowledge, language skills, or current concentration level.	3a. Eliminate unnecessary complexity. 3b. Be consistent with user expectations and intuition. 3c. Accommodate a wide range of literacy and language skills. 3d. Arrange information consistent with its importance. 3e. Provide effective prompting and feedback during and after task completion.
Principle 4: Perceptible Information The design communicates necessary information effectively to the user, regardless of ambient conditions or the user's sensory abilities.	4a. Use different modes (pictorial, verbal, tactile) for redundant presentation of essential information. 4b. Provide adequate contrast between essential information and its surroundings. 4c. Maximize "legibility" of essential information. 4d. Differentiate elements in ways that can be described (i.e., make it easy to give instructions or directions). 4e. Provide compatibility with a variety of techniques or devices used by people with sensory limitations.

Principle 5: Tolerance for Error The design minimizes hazards and the adverse consequences of accidental or unintended actions.	5a. Arrange elements to minimize hazards and errors: most used elements, most accessible; hazardous elements eliminated, isolated, or shielded. 5b. Provide warnings of hazards and errors. 5c. Provide failsafe features. 5d. Discourage unconscious action in tasks that require vigilance.
Principle 6: Low Physical Effort The design can be used efficiently and comfortably and with a minimum of fatigue.	6a. Allow users to maintain a neutral body position. 6b. Use reasonable operating forces. 6c. Minimize repetitive actions. 6d. Minimize sustained physical effort.
Principle 7: Size and Space for Approach and Use Appropriate size and space are provided for approach, reach, manipulation, and use regardless of the user's body size, posture, or mobility.	7a. Provide a clear line of sight to important elements for any seated or standing user. 7b. Make reach to all components comfortable for any seated or standing user. 7c. Accommodate variations in hand and grip size. 7d. Provide adequate space for the use of assistive devices or personal assistance.

Source: (Center for Universal Design, 1997).

be adopted when making considerations for aging in place, and there are several basic design strategies that, if implemented, are likely to ensure that homes are safe, appropriate places for administering healthcare in the home.

The most basic strategy for ensuring individuals can age in place is ensuring that sleeping, bathroom, and kitchen spaces are on an accessible floor level, preferably the first floor (Steinfeld & Maisel, 2012). The ability to seamlessly navigate between these spaces is also crucial. While wider hallways and doorways would be ideal for those in wheelchairs and motorized chairs, homes can be relatively small and affordable while also allowing for an age-in-place approach. Another strategy includes ensuring that outlets, switches, and controls are mounted at an accessible height on the walls. These features should not be too high that those in wheelchairs cannot reach them or too low that individuals have to stoop and risk falling when they need to access them. Lighting is also an important consideration for aging in place. A mixture of overhead and task lighting, placed in strategic places and with easy-to-access controls, allows individuals the autonomy to remain in their homes well into their later years. Including adaptable features like lever-style door knobs, stair lifts, and smart home technologies that allow for communication between cellular phones and a growing market of smart appliances, devices, and sensors can also ensure that individuals avoid unnecessary risks while aging in place (UDS Foundation, 2020).

Preventing Falls

The biggest concern for aging in place is falls. A quarter of U.S. adults aged 65 or older suffer falls each year, which leads to more serious health problems that may prematurely end an individual's tenure in their home of choice (National Institutes of Health [NIH], 2022a). One large barrier to aging in place is the manner in which homes are elevated above the ground plane. Building homes with the slab at grade or altering homes to have no-step entries would prevent falls, which is a major concern for those who are elderly, frail, infirm, or physically disabled. Another cause of falls is uneven or slippery flooring. Installing nonslip, smooth flooring materials and avoiding transitions in the flooring between rooms and spaces could reduce the number of opportunities that may cause falls. Advancements in construction and building materials have produced a wide variety of strategies for installing unobtrusive handrails that individuals can hold on to to help them navigate their home spaces. Patients who have recently lost full mobility will often be provided an in-home physical therapist who helps patients develop strategies for navigating their homes and for falling in a manner that prevents worse injuries. Additionally, assistive and emergency alert technologies could mean the difference between life and death to those who are aging or healing in the home. If a fall were to occur, these technologies alert the appropriate individuals or medical emergency services, without much, or in some cases any, effort by the patient. Avoiding the use of rugs and slippery floor-cleaning products could also help with avoiding falls. These design features are helpful for facilitating this care practice.

A 2015 study of falls among older adults that resulted in emergency department visits found that the most common locations for falls were the bathrooms, bedrooms, and stairs (Moreland et al., 2020). Bathrooms are high-risk spaces for falls, as they require navigating surfaces that are slippery. The risk for falls in bathroom spaces could be mitigated by renovating these spaces with accessible features like grab bars, bench seating, and detachable shower heads and replacing tubs with roll-in showers (Steinfeld & Maisel, 2012). For bedrooms, assistive devices and cellular phones within easy reach, night lights, beds that aren't too high, and discontinuing the use of rugs or other tripping hazards can help. Ensuring that utensils and household tools are easy to reach is likely to help prevent falls in kitchens and utility spaces. Older adults should avoid using stairs, if possible, but should ensure that there are handrails on both sides of all stairways and adequate lighting over stair treads if they must (National Institutes of Health [NIH], 2022b). Healthcare equipment and medical devices are often a necessary component of in-home health care, so the placement and potential hazards of this equipment and medical devices should be considered.

Renovation of Existing Residences for In-Home Care

There are several considerations to ensure adequate renovation of residential homes for in-home care. Input and collaboration with care teams could be highly beneficial for patients, ensuring adequate intervention during hospital visits and after discharge. These teams usually consist of various clinicians and healthcare professionals who perform three types of functions. These functions could be supplementary functions such as injections, complementary functions like those addressing behavioral change, and substitute functions that lean toward diagnosis or treatment (Wagner, 2000). Depending on the health issues of the patient, the team may also include nurses, occupational therapists, physical therapists, speech-language therapists, and social workers (Ellenbecker et al., 2008). The team works together to plan treatment, engage in clinical management, navigate complex treatment protocols, provide educational interventions for self or family management, and coordinate patient follow-ups to mitigate problems that may occur. This approach has proven to be effective for patients with chronic illnesses as well as those who will experience significant changes in the activities of daily living (ADLs) after hospitalization.

The rising need for in-home health care, however, has widened the scope of healthcare teams, calling for a more interdisciplinary mix of professionals. The inclusion of architects, designers, and accessibility consultants on care teams can help healthcare professionals and families of patients with decisions regarding changes in the home for optimal results. These individuals can assist with setting the programmatic needs for home renovations, prioritizing solutions to accessibility issues that are challenges to patients transitioning to in-home care, and providing visualizations that allow the team to understand those challenges in situ. Design professionals possess an interactive expertise that could bring sophistication to the solutions that care teams devise for patients (Kasali & Nersessian, 2015). These professionals are also adept at gathering the input of multiple stakeholders within a project, conducting workshops that could assist with ensuring that design decisions are inclusive and comprehensive.

Another consideration is the facilitation of construction during renovations and relocation of patients if extensive changes are needed. Construction is a messy process, and renovation of existing facilities comes with numerous risks to one's health. One such risk is that the renovation of existing homes could lead to asbestos disturbance, especially if these homes were built during the housing boom and into the 1970s (Park et al., 2013). Abatement can be carried out if asbestos is detected in the home; however, it is found in many parts of the home and can be missed. The presence of construction debris, dust, and vapors could likewise compromise air quality (Racine, 2010). The air quality in homes undergoing renovation could be detrimental to the health of those with existing conditions, not to mention exposing already compromised patients to diseases like mesothelioma (Noonan, 2017). Home renovation projects also come with other hazards that could make navigating and addressing healthcare in the home difficult. Tripping hazards from building waste, periods without power, and the interruption of timely deliveries could be detrimental to the progress of patients requiring in-home care. Care teams with this insight could plan accordingly, ensuring that patients have provisions for care during the renovation process and before transition into the home. Another consideration is the installation of infrastructure for information, communicative, and assistive technologies. If this is considered during the design process, these technologies could keep care teams informed of progress, allowing for a more informed in-home care process (Cogollor et al., 2018). There are also emerging technologies for in-home health care that designers could consider to keep providers informed and address problems when they arise. The limitations of off-the-shelf devices that patients can wear are expanded by the capabilities of artificial intelligence (AI) technologies, which can help with assessment, mental health, and even understanding the behavioral patterns of patients. These devices collect data and parse it for easy consumption by healthcare professionals. These technologies can also be found in the form of apps that work with the devices that patients already own, tracking their progress and communicating health information instantly (Moon et al., 2019). While the capabilities of AI technologies are still being discovered, it is obvious that they have multiple applications for the successful delivery of in-home care. The cost of renovation and installation of the aforementioned technologies is another obvious barrier to consider when considering in-home healthcare; this aspect deserves further consideration, especially considering the limited number of accessible residential spaces available to those who need them.

Conclusion

As evidenced in this chapter, facilitating an effective in-home healthcare process comes with a number of challenges. Addressing these challenges, however, no matter how difficult, can ensure that while the capacity of healthcare facilities and the stock of accessible homes are limited, there are ways to ensure an inclusive healthcare experience for all. Healthcare providers and teams should consider constructing care teams with design professionals that could ensure there is a synergy between established patient care plans and the spaces they will inhabit. While many of the considerations found in this chapter specifically address the aging-in-place approach, these considerations are applicable to a wide variety of issues plaguing patients of all ages and with a variety of health issues. Avoiding stigmas, protecting the autonomy of patients, and considering the role of universal design in the facilitation of healthcare delivery are crucial to ensure that all patients feel valued.

References

Caplan, Z., & Rabe, M. (2023). *The older population: 2020.* Retrieved June 17, 2023, from https://www2.census.gov/library/publications/decennial/2020/census-briefs/c2020br-07.pdf

Centers for Disease Control and Prevention. (n.d.). *COVID data tracker.* Retrieved June 17, 2023, from https://covid.cdc.gov/covid-data-tracker/#hospital-capacity

Center for Universal Design. (1997). *The principles of universal design.* Retrieved June 17, 2023, from https://design.ncsu.edu/wp-content/uploads/2022/11/principles-of-universal-design.pdf

Cogollor, J. M., Rojo-Lacal, J., Hermsdörfer, J., Ferre, M., Arredondo Waldmeyer, M. T., Giachritsis, C., Armstrong, A., Breñosa Martinez, J. M., Bautista Loza, D. A., & Sebastián, J. M. (2018). Evolution of cognitive rehabilitation after stroke from traditional techniques to smart and personalized home-based information and communication technology systems: Literature review. *JMIR Rehabilitation and Assistive Technologies,* 5(1). https://doi.org/10.2196/rehab.8548

Ellenbecker, C. H., Samia, L., Cushman, M. J., & Alster, K. (2008). *Chapter 13: Patient safety and quality in home health care.* Retrieved June 17, 2023, from www.ncbi.nlm.nih.gov/books/NBK2631/pdf/Bookshelf_NBK2631.pdf

Kasali, A., & Nersessian, N. J. (2015). Architects in interdisciplinary contexts: Representational practices in healthcare design. *Design Studies,* 41, 205–223. https://doi.org/10.1016/j.destud.2015.09.001

Moon, J., Lee, K., & Lee, Y. S. (2019). *Integrated system of monitoring and intervention for in-home healthcare and treatment.* Adjunct Proceedings of the 2019 ACM International Joint Conference on Pervasive and Ubiquitous Computing and Proceedings of the 2019 ACM International Symposium on Wearable Computers. https://doi.org/10.1145/3341162.3349313

Moreland, B. L., Kakara, R., Haddad, Y. K., Shakya, I., & Bergen, G. (2020). A descriptive analysis of location of older adult falls that resulted in emergency department visits in the United States, 2015. *American Journal of Lifestyle Medicine,* 15(6), 590–597. https://doi.org/10.1177/1559827620942187

National Institutes of Health (NIH). (2022a, September 12). *Falls and fractures in older adults: Causes and prevention.* Retrieved June 17, 2023, from www.nia.nih.gov/health/falls-and-fractures-older-adults-causes-and-prevention

National Institutes of Health (NIH). (2022b). *Preventing falls at home: Room by room.* National Institute on Aging. www.nia.nih.gov/health/preventing-falls-home-room-room

National Low Income Housing Coalition (NLIHC). (2023). *The gap: A shortage of affordable rental homes.* Retrieved June 17, 2023, from https://nlihc.org/gap

Noonan, C. W. (2017). Environmental asbestos exposure and risk of mesothelioma. *Annals of Translational Medicine,* 5(11), 234–234. https://doi.org/10.21037/atm.2017.03.7b4

Park, E., Yates, D. H., Hyland, R. A., & Johnson, A. R. (2013). Asbestos exposure during home renovation in New South Wales. *Medical Journal of Australia*, 199(6), 410–413. https://doi.org/10.5694/mja12.11802

Racine, W. P. (2010). Emissions concerns during renovation in the healthcare setting: Asbestos abatement of floor tile and mastic in medical facilities. *Journal of Environmental Management*, 91(7), 1429–1436. https://doi.org/10.1016/j.jenvman.2010.02.027

Song, J., Zolnoori, M., McDonald, M. V., Barrón, Y., Cato, K., Sockolow, P., Sridharan, S., Onorato, N., Bowles, K. H., & Topaz, M. (2021). Factors associated with timing of the start-of-care nursing visits in home health care. *Journal of the American Medical Directors Association*, 22(11). https://doi.org/10.1016/j.jamda.2021.03.005

Steinfeld, E., & Maisel, J. L. (2012). *Universal design creating inclusive environments*. John Wiley & Sons.

UDS Foundation. (2020, April 15). *A guide to aging in place design*. Retrieved June 17, 2023, from https://udservices.org/aging-in-place-design/

United States Census Bureau. (n.d.). *U.S. and world population clock*. Retrieved June 17, 2023, from www.census.gov/popclock/

U.S. Access Board. (1984). *Uniform federal accessibility standards (UFAS)*. Retrieved June 17, 2023, from www.access-board.gov/aba/ufas.html

U.S. Department of Justice/U.S. Department of Housing and Urban Development. (2008). *Joint statement of the department of housing and urban development and the department of justice: Reasonable accommodations*. Retrieved June 17, 2023, from www.justice.gov/sites/default/files/crt/legacy/2010/12/15/reasonable_modifications_mar08.pdf

Wagner, E. H. (2000). The role of patient care teams in chronic disease management. *BMJ*, 320. https//doi.org/10.1136/bmj.320.7234.569

CHAPTER 12 EXAMPLE

KIWANA T. McCLUNG

A 69-year-old man has made the transition to live with his family after a heart attack, multiple strokes, and other health issues. The family lives in a split-level home, with the front entry, foyer, kitchen, dining room, bedrooms, and bathrooms at ground level and the den/living room, garage, and patio spaces accessible from a lower level. The front and patio entries are both step-up, requiring the navigation of between 6 and 14 inches. The man has limited mobility on the left side of his body, necessitating the use of a cane, walker, wheelchair, and/or motorized chair. He also uses an ankle-foot orthosis (AFO) brace to assist with stability. He has additional health issues, such as age-related macular degeneration, diabetes, chronic obstructive pulmonary disease (COPD), high blood pressure, benign prostatic hyperplasia, and stroke-related peripheral neuropathy, all of which necessitate the need for healthcare professionals periodically visiting the home. Visits with in-home nurses primarily take place in the den/living room areas, while therapy sessions to assist the patient with exercise and adjusting to the ADLs take place in various places in the home.

Improvements made to the home primarily occurred in the bathroom. The tub was removed and bench-seating installed, along with nonslip flooring, grab bars, accessible fixtures, and accessible nooks for easy access to toiletries. Tripping hazards like rugs, loose cords, and transition strips were also removed from the home. Movement between the upper and lower levels requires the patient to navigate two sets of steps with four risers each, between 28 and 30 inches; each set of steps only has railings on one side. All other accessibility measures are additive equipment, such as medical-grade transfer shower benches near the bathroom sink and emergency alert devices in case of a fall.

The patient's adult son has noted several other changes that can be made to improve the patient's ability to remain in the home through the end of life. A ramp could easily be installed/built at the front entry to eliminate the need for the patient to navigate a step when entering and exiting the home; however, the back entry has two full steps, requiring a longer ramp run. There are no handrails in the hallways or bedrooms of the home. These measures, however, are costly and not covered by insurance. Stair lifts are not only obtrusive but also impractical for the home since they would need to navigate only four steps.

When considerations for aging in place are made during the initial design of residential homes, it is much easier to engage universal design strategies, ensuring that features for accessibility at all ages, abilities, and stages of life are integrated into the design of the home. Adaptation is much harder, however, and some residential features, like those found in split-level or even multistory homes, make adaptation difficult and, in some cases, unfeasible. In this example, some changes are able to be made, but the patient still requires the assistance of family or healthcare professionals for navigating certain aspects of the home. Design professionals engaging in the design or renovation of residential homes and units should consider incorporating accessible or universal features to support the aging-in-place approach and in-home healthcare needs.

Part 3

THE FUTURE OF HEALTHCARE AND ALTERNATIVE HEALTHCARE SITUATIONS

13

RENEWABLE ENERGY IN HEALTHCARE AND ENERGY SYSTEMS FOR RESILIENCE

Kari J. Smith

Introduction

The complex, unpredictable, and compound interactions of global health crises make it challenging for healthcare systems to respond effectively. Navigating the healthcare system's challenges requires an awareness of existing gaps to appropriately address the issues and a diverse team of experts to design solutions to adapt as necessary. In the absence of this approach, what is potentially at stake is the loss of life, social disruption, and the collapse of healthcare services (Kruk et al., 2015).

Many of the most promising solutions to global healthcare challenges have deliberately or inadvertently adopted a convergent research approach. In 2016, the U.S. National Science Foundation (NSF) launched funding for convergence research, which seeks to integrate the knowledge of experts from distinct fields to find innovative solutions to societal needs. As Sundstrom et al. note, most convergence research has focused on integration across health science, nanotechnology, biotechnology, and information technology (Sundstrom et al., 2023, p. 1). A convergence research approach

DOI: 10.4324/9781003414902-16

applied to the health-energy nexus could accelerate healthcare research innovations.

Given the evolving healthcare system landscape and pressing need, a more integrated and collaborative framework for the health-energy nexus is necessary. In the report *Energizing Health: Accelerating Electricity Access in Healthcare Facilities: Executive Summary*, the World Health Organization (WHO) advocated for a convergence research approach between the health and energy sectors to "leverage synergies and maximize impact" in recognition that "health and energy actors have often worked in silos" (WHO, 2023, p. xix). As the WHO notes, energy departments and private energy enterprises that are typically responsible for powering healthcare infrastructure have needed more integration of knowledge, methods, or expertise from colleagues working on healthcare system issues (WHO, 2023, p. 11). A more integrated approach would facilitate more significant policy development, infrastructure planning, system financing, technology procurement, and customized energy solutions for healthcare (WHO, 2023, p. 11).

A Convergence Research Approach for Decentralized Renewable Energy Solutions

The current energy consumption pattern in healthcare negatively contributes to healthcare outcomes and the environment. In 2019, the healthcare sector was responsible for 4.4% of global carbon emissions, and the consumption of fossil fuels for energy for healthcare was more than half of the sector's climate footprint (Karliner & Slotterback, 2019). In their research and policy paper, Karliner et al. argue for a climate-smart approach to bolster healthcare resilience in response to the growing global health and climate crises and the establishment of timelines and a framework to transition from fossil fuel energy to decentralized renewable energy (Karliner & Slotterback, 2019, p. 6). Decentralized renewable energy systems that generate and store energy where it will be used rather than sourced from an industrial plant offer advantages, including natural replenishment, indefinite availability, and reduced environmental impact, compared to traditional fossil fuel energy sources. The delivery of quality healthcare services using decentralized renewable energy systems requires consideration of many techno-economic factors, including an analysis of site characteristics such as environmental and climate factors, knowledge of the electrical load needs, the availability of local energy resources, public policies and incentives, and system cost and financial sources (WHO, 2023, p. xxvi). By incorporating decentralized renewable energy sources into healthcare infrastructure, uninterrupted healthcare delivery can be ensured, especially during power failures that are likely to increase due to the accelerating impacts of the climate crisis.

In January 2023, the WHO published a landmark report, *Energizing Health: Accelerating Electricity Access in Healthcare Facilities: Executive Summary*, that provides insights and recommendations on electricity access and "how to accelerate health facility electrification while supporting the transition to clean, sustainable energy systems that improve health and climate outcomes" (WHO, 2023, p. vi). Challenges such as climate change, natural disasters, and increasing energy demands will necessitate healthcare systems to adapt and become more resilient to ensure continuous and reliable healthcare delivery (WHO, 2023, p. 7). While applicable everywhere, decentralized renewable systems offer many benefits for the world's least developed regions, where healthcare systems must prepare differently for healthcare system resilience. Decentralized renewable systems address existing gaps in the reliability of energy sourcing through diversification and allow for greater self-regulation by reducing net-import dependency on fossil fuels, thereby increasing energy security and reducing vulnerability due to price fluctuations and supply chain disruptions.

Reliable electricity is a critical and underrecognized enabler of universal healthcare (WHO, 2023, p. xvii). Worldwide, millions of people rely on healthcare facilities without reliable electricity access or with no electricity access at all (WHO, 2023, p. xii). Additionally, healthcare facilities with electricity access may experience energy supply disruptions and price fluctuations if they rely on fossil fuels for energy sourced from other countries. According to the International Renewable Energy Agency (IRENA), an estimated 80% of the global population relies heavily on fossil fuels imported from other countries (2022). Energy disruption and energy deficiency are particularly concerning for healthcare facilities requiring a continuous and reliable energy supply to provide essential healthcare. A transition to decentralized renewable energy systems offers a viable energy source to support continuous healthcare delivery. It will play a crucial role in shaping the future of healthcare, particularly in the least developed regions of the world (WHO, 2023, p. xvii).

Decentralized renewable energy systems for healthcare in the least developed regions ensure a more sustainable energy source and address electricity disparities that impact vulnerable populations. Convergence researchers in disaster, healthcare, and decentralized renewable energy solutions advocate for recognizing issues of power and justice embedded in socio-technical-ecological systems (WHO, 2023, p. 40). Ahlborg et al. (2019) highlight the importance of addressing social and environmental inequities in designing and implementing healthcare and energy solutions. A principled approach ensures that the benefits of resilience initiatives are accessible and equitable for all communities. Healthcare system resilience must prioritize inclusivity, fairness, and long-term sustainability while addressing global health and prosperity challenges. A convergence framework approach, as discussed in the context of hazards and disaster research by Lori Peek et al. (2020), further highlights the need for an ethical approach. Peek et al. stress the importance of involving historically underrepresented groups in research.

The authors state:

> This will help ensure that diverse perspectives and paradigms are brought to bear to respond to pressing challenges through elevating research outcomes designed to promote collective well-being.
>
> (Peek et al., 2020, p. 2)

A diverse research team often leads to a broader range of ideas and insights, ensuring that the solutions developed are equitable and effective for all communities, particularly those vulnerable or marginalized. Furthermore, this approach ensures that the threats identified and specific actions to address the problem can reduce historical inequities and injustices that exacerbate hazards into disasters (Peek et al., 2020). Similarly, researchers in socio-technical-ecological systems (Ahlborg et al., 2019) and decentralized renewable energy solutions are interested in justice approaches to empower rural communities, low-income populations, and those without political clout or governance.

Emilio Moran et al. insist:

> it is essential to change the top-down paradigm often found in development programs, and instead use an approach in which scientists work with community members experiencing these challenges firsthand in solving their problems.
>
> (Moran et al., 2022)

Adding to the definition and framework of healthcare resilience, the often-cited article by Margaret Kruk et al., written after the Ebola crisis, states:

"Health systems are resilient if they protect human life and produce good health outcomes for all during a crisis and its aftermath" (Kruk et al., 2015, p. 1910). Resilient health systems can also deliver everyday benefits and positive health outcomes. This double benefit – improved performance in both bad times and good – is what has been called 'the resilience dividend.'

(Kruk et al., 2015, p. 1910)

Researchers at the Massachusetts Institute of Technology (MIT) (2016) recognized that a convergence framework is not the panacea for solving the severe challenges of the healthcare system, but it is a pathway to progress and innovation. A forward-looking pathway informed by the insights of past failures and an understanding of the multiplicity of preconditions that may compromise the healthcare system offer an alternative approach to the dominant current practice.

Examples

Organizations with dynamic approaches seeking to blend diverse knowledge, methods, and expertise across multiple fields, like the United Nations Development Programme (UNDP), exemplify specific projects. These initiatives showcase the NSF's conceptualization of a convergence framework that addresses problems emerging from critical healthcare system needs. The UNDP is a global development network that advocates for change and connects countries to knowledge, experience, and resources to help people build a better life. The agency emphasizes developing local capacity toward long-term self-sufficiency and prosperity and has created and promoted an environment that enables research, innovation, and learning.

One of the primary goals of the UNDP is to support sustainable development worldwide. The United Nations Sustainable Development Goals (SDGs) are a call for action "to promote prosperity while protecting the planet" (Neshovski, n.d.). Decentralized renewable energy use in healthcare aligns with several SDGs, including Goal 3: Good Health and Well-being, Goal 7: Affordable and Clean Energy, and Goal 13: Climate Action. Many healthcare facilities, particularly those in remote and underserved areas, face challenges with reliable access to electricity. By funding decentralized renewable energy system projects, the UNDP helps improve energy access in these regions, ensuring that healthcare services can be delivered effectively and consistently.

The UNDP is involved in various projects, conceptualized and implemented, from the scale of facilities to specialized equipment, that promote decentralized renewable and alternative energy systems solutions in healthcare settings worldwide. In areas where the primary power grid is not accessible to all, is unreliable, or is insufficient, the UNDP has supported the development of microgrids that incorporate decentralized renewable energy sources. Solar and wind systems, combined with energy storage systems, are a source of essential electricity for lighting, medical equipment, and refrigeration for vaccines and medications. In other regions, the UNDP has supported sustainable biomass projects that utilize agricultural waste or locally sourced biomass to generate energy for healthcare facilities. The UNDP has also explored the use of geothermal energy for heating and cooling healthcare facilities. At the equipment scale, the UNDP has facilitated the deployment of solar-powered vaccine refrigerators. These refrigerators ensure that vaccines are stored at the right temperature, even during power outages, maintaining their effectiveness and potency. The UNDP has also implemented projects to improve healthcare buildings' energy efficiency by retrofitting existing healthcare facilities with energy-efficient lighting, heating, cooling, and insulation to reduce energy consumption and environmental impact. The UNDP recognizes that using decentralized renewable energy systems to support continuous healthcare delivery offers numerous benefits and advantages (Energy and Health |United Nations Development Programme, n.d.) An additional case study analysis in India, Uganda, and Nepal of healthcare facility electrification realized using a convergence research approach can be found in the WHO's report *Energizing Health: Accelerating Electricity Access in Healthcare Facilities: Executive Summary* (2023).

The WHO reports that reliable electricity is crucial to providing better healthcare outcomes, including reduced mortality through prenatal and newborn care (WHO, 2023, p. 3). The author and a transdisciplinary team of experienced investigators and consultants from diverse disciplines utilized a convergence framework to address a maternal-infant health and wellness challenge in disaster preparedness and disaster response planning – the need for private and sanitary spaces for lactating mothers and their infants to breastfeed or lactating mothers to express.

Our response aimed to bridge a significant gap in disaster preparedness and response planning concerning health and wellness, thereby reducing the negative impacts of the most vulnerable in rural communities by promoting postdisaster security and access to safe spaces. The team developed a patented portable location unit as a disaster response and recovery solution that enabled emergency organizations and the private/business sector to address the vital feeding needs of children under two years old and lactating women in postdisaster situations (2021). The solution sought to minimize infant and young child morbidity and maximize infant and young child nutrition, health, and development. A project of this complexity required a diverse team to address the multitude of design issues, best practices, and regulations necessary to develop the solution. The team consisted of experts with prior transdisciplinary research records; postdisaster recovery experience; patient outcome, evidence-based maternal and infant care practice; product and empathy design training; sustainable habitat design experience; innovation and technical acuity; business acumen; and intellectual property proficiency.

Natural hazards may, and natural disasters do, disrupt everyday life and can have significant adverse health effects on affected populations, particularly in rural areas. "Resource-constrained settings" (WHO, 2023, p. xxv), such as postdisaster rural areas, require improved energy system healthcare-resilient solutions to ensure reliable and sustainable power supply to serve vulnerable populations (WHO, 2023, p. 10). A climate-resilient healthcare energy source system in these settings is necessary, given the increased frequency and intensity of extreme events associated with climate change that disrupt the electricity supply (WHO, 2023, p. xxvii). Beyond reliable energy, the unpredictable water supply needed for washing, sanitation, and hygiene in postdisaster settings also requires climate-resilient solutions adapted to the evolving risks. Our solution, an easily deployable portable unit equipped with a decentralized renewable energy system coupled with water storage, is energy and water-use efficient and achieves healthcare-standard best practices. The solution is depicted in Figure 13.1.

The disaster emergency management phases of preparedness, response, and recovery are incredibly stressful for lactating women. Unfortunately, most of the disaster planning for lactating mothers focuses on the safe storage of frozen milk supply during evacuation and shelter-in-place recovery

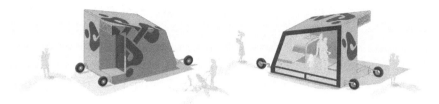

Figure 13.1 Schematic rendering of the U.S. design patented portable lactation unit
(Babin et al., 2021).

rather than the ability of emergency shelters to serve the needs of displaced lactating mothers. As a result, women and infants experience adverse effects. As authors Aros-Vera et al. (2021, p. 2) reported, women in affected areas tend to have lower and shorter breastfeeding rates during natural disasters than the national average. The authors state that factors contributing to shorter breastfeeding rates in postdisaster settings include inadequate privacy for breastfeeding, maternal misconceptions about breastfeeding production and milk quality, and maternal confidence in breastfeeding during crises (Aros-Vera et al., 2021, p. 2). Even in nondisaster settings, the national breastfeeding rates remain below the recommendations of the American Academy of Pediatrics and other U.S. health organizations, especially among participants in the Special Supplemental Nutrition Program for Women, Infants, and Children (WIC).

A case for the economic benefits of our portable lactation unit included a justification of the potential cost savings for WIC and Medicaid. WIC, a federally funded program, provides supplemental foods, healthcare referrals, and nutrition education for low-income pregnant, breastfeeding, and nonbreastfeeding postpartum women and infants and children up to age five who are at nutritional risk (Department of Labor, n.d.). In 2019, Oliveira, Prell, and Cheng reported to Congress that increasing breastfeeding rates in WIC households to medically recommended levels could lead to significant cost savings, totaling around $9.1 billion. Medical costs would make up $1.5 billion of these savings, while nonmedical costs would contribute another $0.6 billion. Most savings, approximately $6.9 billion, would result from a reduction in early deaths, comprising over three-quarters of the estimated cost savings associated with higher breastfeeding rates in WIC

(Oliveira et al., 2019). With a focus on protecting, promoting, and supporting breastfeeding in emergencies, the project would enable federal and state emergency response agencies and community health workers to address vital infant feeding needs in postdisaster situations to improve community health outcomes.

Conclusion

The WHO has identified that climate change is our century's most significant global health threat and will continue to strain the healthcare system and most negatively impact those least capable of adapting (WHO, 2023, p. 6). A solution with broad consensus is that healthcare systems should adapt to decentralized renewable energy to advance positive healthcare and environmental and climate outcomes (WHO, 2023, p. 44). While many barriers exist to the adaptation of decentralized renewable and alternative energy systems in healthcare systems, such as technical procurement, institutional capacity, policy constraints, and financing barriers, the WHO believes that these can be surmounted through more significant political commitment and leadership to ensure advocacy, mainstreaming, monitoring, and accountability (WHO, 2023, xxxiv).

A convergence research approach presents a promising pathway to bridge the gap between existing barriers and a vision for a decentralized renewable energy system for a healthcare system. NSF Director Sethuraman Panchanathan highlighted in his October 21, 2022, presentation, "Innovation Anywhere, Opportunities Everywhere: Accelerating the Frontiers of Science and Technology," that dismantling funding barriers and fostering an inclusive research approach can unlock innovation potential. A convergent research approach offers a revolutionary way to enhance healthcare energy resilience and is a necessity for the well-being of the planet and its inhabitants.

Acknowledgements

ChatGPT was used in the preparation of this chapter to conduct background research on UNDP's projects. The original AI output was verified using UNDP's reports, and the author adapted and modified the text while writing the chapter.

References

Ahlborg, H., Ruiz-Mercado, I., Molander, S., & Masera, O. (2019). Bringing technology into social-ecological systems research – motivations for a socio-technical-ecological systems approach. *Sustainability, 11*(7), 2009. https://doi.org/10.3390/su11072009

Aros-Vera, F., Chertok, I. R. A., & Melnikov, S. (2021, November). Emergency and disaster response strategies to support mother-infant dyads during COVID-19. *International Journal of Disaster Risk Reduction, 65,* 102532. https://doi.org/10.1016/j.ijdrr.2021.102532; Epub August 25, 2021. PMID: 34458086; PMCID: PMC8386097.

Babin, B., Boudreaux, S., Hurst, H., Lemoine, J., & Smith, K. (2021, February 16). *Portable lactation & women's health unit (US D910,873 S)*. United States Patent and Trademark Office. www.uspto.gov/

Department of Labor. (n.d.). *Federal resources for women*. U.S. Department of Labor – Women's Bureau. https://www.dol.gov/agencies/wb/federal-agency-resources

Energy and Health | United Nations Development Programme. (n.d.). UNDP. Retrieved October 10, 2023, from www.undp.org/energy/our-work-areas/energy-and-health

IEA. (2021). *Recommendations of the global commission on people-centered clean energy transitions*. IEA. www.iea.org/reports/recommendations-of-the-global-commission-on-people-centred-clean-energy-transitions. License: CC BY 4.0.

IEA. (2022). *SDG7: Data and projections*. IEA. www.iea.org/reports/sdg7-data-and-projections. License: CC BY 4.0.

Karliner, J., & Slotterback, S. (2019). *Health care's climate footprint: How the health sector contributes to the global climate crisis and opportunities for action. Health care without harm climate-smart health care series Green Paper number one produced in collaboration with Arup.* https://noharm-global.org/sites/default/files/documents-files/5961/HealthCaresClimateFootprint_092319.pdf

Kruk, M. E., Myers, M. D., Varpilah, S. T., & Dahn, B. (2015). What is a resilient health system? Lessons from Ebola. *The Lancet, 385.* https://doi.org/10.1016/s0140-6736(15)60755-3

Moran, E. F., Lopez, M. C., Mourão, R., Brown, E., McCright, A. M., Walgren, J., Bortoleto, A. P., Mayer, A., Johansen, I. C., Ramos, K. N., Castro-Diaz, L., Garcia, M. A., Lembi, R. C., & Mueller, N. (2022, December 6). Advancing convergence research: Renewable energy solutions for off-grid communities. *Proceedings of the National Academy of Sciences, 119*(49), e2207754119. https//doi.org/10.1073/pnas.2207754119; Epub November 28, 2022. PMID: 36442126; PMCID: PMC9897475.

Neshovski, R. (n.d.). Home. United Nations Sustainable Development. www.un.org/sustainabledevelopment/#:~:text=The%20Sustainable%20Development%20Goals%20are

Oliveira, V., Prell, M., & Cheng, X. (2019, February). *The economic impacts of breastfeeding: A focus on USDA's special supplemental nutrition program for women, infants, and children (WIC), ERR-261.* U.S. Department of Agriculture, Economic Research Service.

Peek, L., Tobin, J., Adams, R. M., Wu, H., & Mathews, M. C. (2020). A framework for convergence research in the hazards and disaster field: The natural hazards engineering research infrastructure converge facility. *Frontiers Built Environment, 6,* 110. https//doi.org/10.3389/fbuil.2020.00110

Sundstrom, S. M., Angeler, D. G., Ernakovich, J. G., García, J. H., Hamm, J. A., Huntington, O., & Allen, C. R. (2023). The emergence of convergence. *Elementa: Science of the Anthropocene, 11*(1). https://doi.org/10.1525/elementa.2022.00128

United Nations. (n.d.). *Renewable energy — powering a safer future*. United Nations. www.un.org/en/climatechange/raising-ambition/renewable-energy#:~:text=About%2080%20percent%20of%20the

World Health Organization (WHO). (2023, October 3). *Energizing health: Accelerating electricity access in health-care facilities: Executive summary*. World Health Organization. Switzerland. https://policycommons.net/artifacts/3370601/energizing-health/4169266/. CID: 20.500.12592/mtjnrb.

14

INNOVATIONS IN HEALTHCARE DESIGN

DEVICE, DELIVERY, AND SYSTEM

Elham Morshedzadeh

What does innovation mean in the healthcare industry? This question can be answered from many different points of view. According to the World Health Organization (WHO), health innovation is described as a novel or enhanced solution that can greatly improve positive health outcomes. The WHO's Innovation Scaling Framework exemplifies their collaborative approach to expanding the use and impact of innovation, which involves three key dimensions. This first requires an understanding of the health demands and priorities of different countries. The second ensures a sufficient supply of innovations are ready for large-scale implementation. Last, the framework emphasizes the importance of continuous assessment throughout the entire process – from incubation of new innovations through partners to effective implementation and sustainability. This multipartner approach enables WHO to effectively address the challenges and complexities associated with scaling innovations within the healthcare sector (WHO, 2023).

In recent years, the healthcare industry has undergone a remarkable wave of innovations that are reshaping the delivery of healthcare, transforming

DOI: 10.4324/9781003414902-17

not only patient care but also the new vision toward healthcare workers and related communities. These innovations are driven by a range of factors, including advancements in technology, evolving patient needs and conditions, new discoveries in disease and/or medical conditions, and even topics such as environmental changes and their impact on health. The common goal across the expanse of these innovations, however, is to enhance access to care, improve patient outcomes, and optimize healthcare operations. The focus is on developing solutions that can address the challenges and complexities of the healthcare system, ultimately leading to better healthcare experiences and improved health outcomes for patients.

Patient-Centered Design and Its Impact on Healthcare

Research concerning new frontiers in healthcare innovation reveal various emerging areas with connection to education, science, technology (Lee & Yoon, 2021), or a combination of these three.

Industrial designers traditionally have been a part of medical device design and innovation teams for world-renowned companies such as Johnson & Johnson, Philips, General Electric, Stryker, etc. (Proclinical, 2022). The evolving role of designers in healthcare has shifted from providing user-friendly and functionable design that is appropriate to engineers and manufacturer's needs to now prioritizing patient-centered research and design. Patient-centered design is a healthcare design model adopted from user-centered design (UCD) (Rodriguez et al., 2007). The UCD process is a holistic and widely embraced methodology utilized by designers across various specialized fields, including product design, user experience design, interaction design, and web design, among others. At its core, this approach revolves around the fundamental philosophy of empathizing with the user throughout the design process, ensuring that their requirements and needs are met effectively. By focusing on users in design decisions, UCD aims to create solutions that enhance the user experience and deliver optimal outcomes (DIN, 1999; Sanchez Antelo et al., 2022).

The UCD approach has been utilized in many fields such as business, industry, entrepreneurship, economy, sociology, and education, just to name a few; assuredly, the fields of healthcare and the healthcare systems are not an exception to this. For example, Stanford Biodesign is a program at Stanford University that focuses on fostering innovation and entrepreneurship in biomedical technology with a user-focused approach (Stanford Byers Center for Biodesign, 2024). This program brings together interdisciplinary teams of engineers, designers, physicians, and business professionals to identify unmet healthcare needs and develop solutions to address them.

User engagement and participation are the key elements of UCD involving users throughout the entire design process, from research to adoption and diffusion, to create solutions that meet their needs effectively (Hernandez, 2013). In healthcare, the initial step of adopting UCD as patient-centered design involves patient engagement and participation. Patient-reported outcomes (PROs) play a vital role in assessing the effects of medical devices on patient outcomes and promoting patient-centered design. PROs are measures that capture patients' perspectives on their own health status, symptoms, and quality of life. By directly engaging patients in the assessment process, PROs provide valuable insights into the real-world impact of medical devices on patients' lives (U.S. Food and Drug, 2009; Coens et al., 2020; Gnanasakthy et al., 2019). They offer a comprehensive understanding of patient experiences, treatment effectiveness, and quality of care, going beyond traditional clinical measures (Flythe, 2020). Incorporating PROs in the evaluation of medical devices enables a more patient-centered approach to healthcare, ensuring that devices are designed and optimized to meet patients' needs and improve their well-being. By prioritizing patient perspectives and outcomes, the use of PROs facilitates more-informed decision-making, fosters patient empowerment, and contributes to the development of more effective and patient-centric medical devices.

By placing patients, their connection with other stakeholders, and their communities at the center of the innovation process, healthcare organizations and researchers can gain valuable insights into patients' needs, preferences, and experiences, leading to more sustainable solutions. This patient-centric approach helps to identify gaps in current healthcare provisions and drives development toward more effective and patient-centric innovations. Patient-centered research encourages collaboration between healthcare providers, researchers, and patients, fostering a multidisciplinary approach that considers diverse perspectives (Hirsch, 2019). This collaboration leads to the creation of innovative solutions that address real-world challenges and improve patient outcomes. Additionally, patient-centered design ensures that healthcare innovations are tailored to meet the unique needs of individuals, subsequently enhancing their experience and satisfaction with healthcare services. Ultimately, the integration of patient-centered research and design into healthcare innovation contributes to the development of more personalized, efficient, and patient-centered healthcare solutions. This can be achieved using established UCD methods such as interviews, questionnaires, focus groups, and participatory design processes by interdisciplinary teams that include healthcare professionals, community experts, representatives, and designers.

Several successful patient-centered design initiatives have been implemented in healthcare settings, displaying the positive impact of putting patients at the center of the design process. One notable example is the OpenNotes project, which involved sharing clinical notes and visiting summaries with patients through online portals (Walker et al., 2019). This initiative was aimed at enhancing transparency, patient engagement, and shared decision-making. Studies have shown that patients who have access to their medical notes report feeling more in control of their healthcare and have a better understanding of their health conditions (Esch, 2016; Mishra et al., 2019; Walker et al., 2019). Another successful initiative is the Planetree model, which focuses on humanizing healthcare environments and fostering a patient-centered culture (Luzzi, 2021). It emphasizes patient empowerment, holistic care, and the integration of mind, body, and spirit. Facilities implementing the Planetree model have seen improvements in patient satisfaction, staff engagement, and health outcomes (Bogaert, 2022; Lauer, 2021). In the field of medical device design, there are examples like the Empatica Embrace wearable device. This device was specifically designed for individuals with epilepsy, allowing for patient monitoring and providing alerts to the caregivers when seizures occur. By involving patients and caregivers in the design process, Empatica created a device that not only addresses their specific needs but also enhances their quality of life and safety (McCarthy, 2016). The Stanford Medicine 25 initiative is another successful patient-centered design effort focused on teaching healthcare providers how to effectively communicate with patients through bedside diagnostic skills (The Stanford Medicine 25, n.d.). This initiative emphasizes the importance of empathy, patient-centered communication, and physical examination skills, leading to improved diagnostic accuracy and stronger patient-provider relationships (Balogh, 2015; Chi, 2016). These examples demonstrate that patient-centered design initiatives can lead to tangible benefits in healthcare settings. Incorporating patient perspectives, preferences, and needs into the design process has resulted in enhanced patient experiences, improved outcomes, and a shift toward a more patient-centered healthcare system.

Healthcare Innovation and the Changing Landscape

Healthcare innovation is an ever-evolving field driven by the continuous advancements in technology, evolving patient needs, and the ongoing pursuit of improved healthcare outcomes. The landscape of healthcare is currently undergoing significant transformations, influenced by several key factors that are shaping the direction of innovation. Collaboration and partnerships play a crucial role in healthcare innovation due to the inherent complexity of healthcare challenges. This necessitates the stakeholders from various domains work collaboratively; these stakeholders include healthcare providers, technology companies, researchers, policy makers, and patient advocacy groups. These efforts facilitate the sharing of knowledge, harness diverse expertise, and drive innovation, incorporating insights from different perspectives.

In addition to collaboration, other major factors are shaping the future of healthcare innovation. One major driver in this area is an increased focus on personalized medicine. Contemporary understanding of genetic factors, molecular biology, and biomarkers has paved the way for targeted therapies and precision medicine approaches (Minvielle, 2014). Regarding personalization and customization in design for healthcare, medical devices can be tailored to specific patient requirements, ensuring optimal fit, comfort, and effectiveness, ultimately providing more healthcare equity (Jin, 2022). This approach acknowledges the diversity among patients and recognizes that a one-size-fits-all approach is not suitable for everyone (Kim, 2020). Customization in medical device design allows for personalized solutions that enhance patient outcomes, improve user experience, and promote patient satisfaction. It enables healthcare professionals to address individual variations, anatomical differences, and specific medical conditions, leading to better treatment outcomes and improved quality of life for patients (Minvielle, 2021).

Another significant aspect of healthcare innovation is the integration of digital technologies. The rise of digital health solutions, including telemedicine, mobile health apps, wearable devices, and electronic health records, has revolutionized healthcare delivery and patient engagement (Savage, 2018).

Designing these novel interventions, in addition to incorporating engineering and medical knowledge, requires meticulous user research employing UCD methodologies (as previously discussed). This process encompasses usability evaluation, user experience analysis, and, in the case of devices integrating screens (whether physical or virtual), user journey mapping, user interface design, and user interaction design. Within this context, industrial designers assume a vital position as members of a critical thinking team contributing their specialized knowledge to advancing the objectives of these innovations (Al-Daraghmeh, 2022). These technologies enable remote monitoring, virtual consultations, personalized health tracking, and access to medical information, empowering individuals to take an active role in their own care.

Artificial intelligence (AI) and machine learning (ML) are transforming healthcare by analyzing vast amounts of data, identifying patterns, and making predictions that aid in diagnosis, treatment planning, and disease management. AI-powered algorithms can sift through medical records, radiological images, and genetic data to provide more accurate and timely diagnoses. Additionally, AI-driven decision support systems enhance clinical decision-making, which can reduce errors and improve patient safety. AI and ML technologies are continuously evolving, demonstrating their potential to revolutionize healthcare delivery across various specialties. AI can significantly impact healthcare equity by addressing disparities in access, quality, and outcomes. AI technologies can also enhance healthcare delivery by improving efficiency, accuracy, and cost-effectiveness. This can help bridge the gap in healthcare disparities, especially for underserved populations who may face barriers accessing quality care. However, it is crucial to ensure that AI algorithms are trained on diverse and representative datasets to mitigate bias and avoid exacerbating existing inequities (Dankwa-Mullan, 2021). Not only including the sources that ensure diversity but also health equity remains as one of the long-term approaches toward ensuring inclusion. It is pertinent for the system to recognize the diversity right at its roots so that everyone involved in the research gets on board (Zou & Schiebinger, 2021). By harnessing the potential of AI while upholding principles of equity, healthcare systems can work toward providing accessible and equitable care for all individuals, regardless of their background or socioeconomic status. (Johnson, 2022). To ensure healthcare equity, design process principles such as co-creating innovative solutions with stakeholders and community engagement can be employed, while AI and data-informed techniques can lead to promoting equitable healthcare for all (Clark, 2021).

Lastly, the changing demographics and epidemiological patterns are shaping healthcare innovation. Aging populations, the increasing prevalence of chronic diseases, wars, immigration, and other global health challenges necessitate innovative solutions to address these complex issues (Flynn, 2014; Guo, 2020; Holeman, 2020; Mostaghel, 2016). Innovations in healthcare delivery, preventive measures, early detection, and disease management are all essential for promoting population health and addressing the changing healthcare needs of individuals and communities. Embracing the innovative possibilities enables healthcare systems to adapt, improve patient outcomes, enhance patient experiences, and create a sustainable, responsive healthcare environment.

Accessible and Equitable Healthcare Design

Accessibility and equity are crucial components of a well-functioning healthcare system, and designing for these aspects can be approached from various points of view. Design for healthcare is complex in nature, and considering equity, fairness, and accessibility can be translated into even more complex design discussions. Although equity can make design more complex since it relates to humans, human interactions, community relations, and emotions, it turns the design process into a relatable and compassionate experience for not only the designers and creators but also the stakeholders and communities involved.

Accessible and equitable healthcare design refers to the creation of healthcare systems, facilities, and services that are inclusive, are barrier-free, and provide equal access and opportunities for all individuals, regardless of their physical, sensory, cognitive, or socioeconomic abilities as well as their racial, religious, and cultural backgrounds. This design approach aims to reduce disparities in healthcare access and ensure that everyone can receive the care they need in a dignified and supportive environment (Tzenios, 2019). Various points of view in accessible and equitable healthcare design are:

- *Physical Equity and Accessibility:* This involves designing healthcare facilities that are accessible to individuals with mobility impairments, such as those who use wheelchairs or have difficulty walking.

- *Sensory Equity and Accessibility*: Healthcare environments should be designed with consideration for individuals with sensory impairments, such as those who are deaf, hard of hearing, or visually impaired. This consideration in design can greatly enhance the experience for these individuals and ensure effective communication with healthcare providers.
- *Cognitive (and Mental) Equity and Accessibility*: This is essential in creating environments and systems that are easily navigable and understandable for individuals with cognitive impairments, learning disabilities, or dementia. This can be achieved through clear signage, simple instructions, visual aids, and minimizing sensory overload. Creating a calm and supportive atmosphere helps reduce anxiety and promotes a positive healthcare experience for all patients.
- *Socioeconomic Equity and Accessibility*: This includes designing healthcare systems and policies for all individuals with diverse socioeconomic backgrounds. For example, support systems can be provided to rural and underserved populations. These support systems include financial assistance programs, community health centers, and appropriate telehealth services.
- *Community-Sensitive Equity and Accessibility*: Cultural and linguistic diversity are considered to ensure that healthcare facilities and services are culturally sensitive and provide language assistance for individuals with limited English proficiency (assuming English is the most used language in that region). This can be achieved through the designs, devices, and systems that are customizable or are designed in collaboration with the community and their representatives, who understand the unique needs and beliefs of diverse patient populations.
- *Unbiased and Nondiscriminatory Accessibility*: Discrimination, bias, and unconscious stereotypes within the healthcare system can lead to unequal treatment and disparities in care. These barriers need to be addressed through cultural competence training and creating an inclusive healthcare environment (Braveman, 2003).

Overall, accessible and equitable healthcare design strives to create healthcare environments and systems that are inclusive, respectful, and responsive to the diverse needs of individuals. This approach can improve healthcare outcomes, enhance patient experiences (patient-centered design), and foster a more just and equitable healthcare system for all. Providing accessible healthcare can lead to economic benefits for individuals and communities. When people have access to affordable and timely healthcare, they are more likely to maintain good health, stay productive, and contribute to the workforce.

Initiatives addressing healthcare disparities and improving access for underserved populations are 1) telehealth and digital health solutions, 2) community health centers, 3) health workforce diversity, 4) targeted health programs, and 5) health education and engagement.

By implementing these initiatives in innovation and design, healthcare systems can make significant progress in addressing disparities, ensuring accessibility, and fostering equitable healthcare for all individuals, regardless of their background or circumstances.

Strategies for Implementing Patient-Centered Design Principles in Healthcare Settings and Delivery

Through thoughtful and inclusive design practices, industrial design has an integral role in building an accessible and equitable healthcare system and the power to create healthcare products, services, and environments that prioritize the needs and experiences of patients and communities. Industrial designers can create solutions that are intuitive, user-friendly, and tailored to diverse populations by investigating user/patient journeys. Also, engaging with community stakeholders, including patients, healthcare providers, and policy makers, enables industrial designers to gain valuable insights into the specific challenges and barriers faced by their intended populations. This approach fosters empathy, cultural competence, and a deep understanding of the social determinants of health for all parties involved. In addition, it creates the opportunity for designers to drive positive change, improving healthcare access and promoting health equity for all. The design process provides key strategies that are implemented and adjusted for this approach, such as:

1. *User Research:* Including data and feedback collection such as interviews, surveys, observations, think tanks and focus groups, data analysis, user persona and journey analysis, pattern discovery, and needs prioritization.
2. *Participatory-Design and Systematic Thinking:* This strategy helps create an effective system for all entities to understand each other and work

together. This collaborative approach fosters shared decision-making and problem-solving and ensures that the final design reflects the input and expertise of those who will use it. It also fosters trust, a culture of empathy, and compassion among communities and their members; strengthens community bonds; and promotes a sense of ownership and pride in the final outcomes.

3. *Iterative Design Process:* Agility in the design process allows continuous participation of the community in improvement and refinement of solutions. Feedback given by the patients and healthcare providers ensures that the designs are responsive to their evolving needs and preferences.

4. *Inclusive and Sustainable Design:* This method uses critical thinking to create accessible and environmentally conscious solutions that cater to diverse needs and minimize negative impacts. It prioritizes inclusivity for all individuals and promotes environmental stewardship. This means establishing a continuous mechanism for system effectiveness, patient satisfaction, health outcomes, and overall experience evaluation of a sustainable ecosystem.

5. *Health Design and Communication:* Communication and educational tools in various formats, such as infographics, diagrams, and interactive media, can simplify complex health information and make it easier for community members to understand and apply in their daily lives. Designing culturally sensitive and inclusive communication materials also helps ensure that health directives reach diverse populations.

Design has the potential to be a catalyst in fostering community engagement and collaboration. The nature of the design process calls for collaboration, compassion, and thinking from another point of view rather than one's own. This method of thinking in healthcare design can lead to improved health outcomes by empowering individuals, enhancing communication, and creating supportive environments, while leveraging technology in an ethical manner. Figure 14.1 visualizes the importance of community engagement in the design process.

Placing the community at the center of the design process can ultimately lead to improved quality of life for all. Healthcare professionals bring their expertise in patient care, medical knowledge, and understanding of healthcare systems. Designers offer their skills in user experience, creative

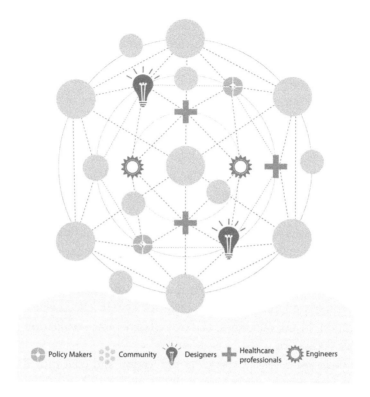

Figure 14.1 Community engagement.

problem-solving, and innovation. Policy makers have the power to create an enabling environment through policies that support accessibility and equity in healthcare. Communities provide valuable insights into their needs, preferences, and experiences. By working in partnership with various allied professionals, we can drive meaningful change in healthcare design and delivery. It is only through our joint efforts and compassionate partnership that innovative designs can break down barriers, eliminate disparities, and support a healthcare system that truly serves and uplifts every individual and community with equal access to high-quality healthcare that meets their unique needs. Figure 14.2 demonstrates the context of various stakeholders in the design process.

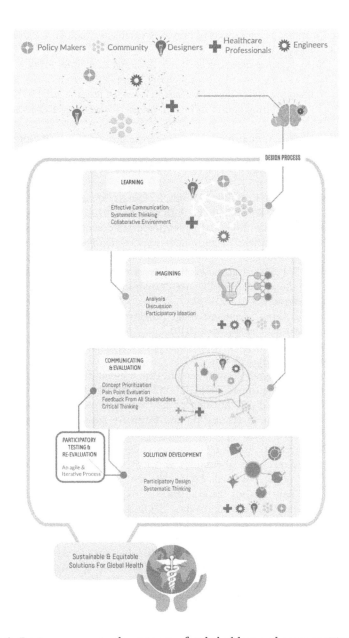

Figure 14.2 Design process in the context of stakeholders and communities.

References

Al-Daraghmeh, M. Y. (2022). A review of medical wearables: Materials, power sources, sensors, and manufacturing aspects of human wearable technologies. Journal of Medical Engineering & Technology, 1–15.

Balogh, E. P. (2015). Improving diagnosis in health care. National Academies Press.

Bogaert, B. (2022). Moving toward person-centered care: Valuing emotions in hospital design and architecture. HERD: Health Environments Research & Design Journal, 15(2), 355–364.

Braveman, P. (2003). Defining equity in health. Journal of Epidemiology & Community Health, 57(4), 254–258.

Chi, J. A. (2016). The five-minute moment. The American Journal of Medicine, 129(8), 792–795.

Clark, C. W. (2021). Health care equity in the use of advanced analytics and artificial intelligence technologies in primary care. Journal of General Internal Medicine, 36, 3188–3193.

Coens, C., Pe, M., Dueck, A. C., Sloan, J., Basch, E., Calvert, M., Bottomley, A., Campbell, A., Cleeland, C., Cocks, K., Collette, L., & Devlin, N. (2020). International standards for the analysis of quality-of-life and patient-reported outcome endpoints in cancer randomised controlled trials: Recommendations of the SISAQOL Consortium. The Lancet Oncology, 21(2), e83–e96.

Dankwa-Mullan, I. S. (2021). A proposed framework on integrating health equity and racial justice into the artificial intelligence development lifecycle. Journal of Health Care for the Poor and Underserved, 32(2), 300–317.

Din, E. (1999). 13407: Human-centered design processes for interactive systems. Brussels, CEN-European Committee for Standardization, 9(10).

Esch, T. M. (2016). Engaging patients through open notes: An evaluation using mixed methods. BMJ Open, 105(4), 798–801.

Flynn, M. A. (2014). Immigration, work, and health: A literature review of immigration between Mexico and the United States. Revista de trabajo Social, 6, 129–149.

Flythe, J. E. (2020). Toward patient-centered innovation: A conceptual framework for patient-reported outcome measures for transformative kidney replacement devices. Clinical Journal of the American Society of Nephrology, 15(10), 1522–1530.

Gnanasakthy, A., Barrett, A., Evans, E., D'Alessio, D., & Romano, C. D. (2019). A review of patient-reported outcomes labeling for oncology drugs approved by the FDA and the EMA (2012–2016). Value in Health, 22(2), 203–209.

Guo, C. A. (2020). Challenges for the evaluation of digital health solutions – a call for innovative evidence generation approaches. NPJ Digital Medicine, 3(1), 110.

Hernandez, S. E.-S. (2013). Patient-centered innovation in health care organizations. Health Care Management Review, 38(2), 166–175.

Hirsch, G. (2019). Leaping together toward sustainable, patient-centered innovation: The value of a multistakeholder safe haven for accelerating system change. Clinical Pharmacology and Therapeutics, 105(4), 798–801.

Holeman, I., & Kane, D. (2020). Human-centered design for global health equity. Information Technology for Development, 26(3), 477–505.

Jin, Z. H. (2022). Balancing the customization and standardization: Exploration and layout surrounding the regulation of the growing field of 3D-printed medical devices in China. Bio-Design and Manufacturing, 5(3), 580–606.

Johnson, A. E. (2022). Utilizing artificial intelligence to enhance health equity among patients with heart failure. *Heart Failure Clinics, 18*(2), 259–273.

Kim, N. W. (2020). A customized smart medical mask for healthcare personnel. In *IEEE international conference on industrial engineering and engineering management (IEEM)* (pp. 581–585). IEEE.

Lauer, J. (2021). *Planetree model and improving patient care outcomes.* Misericordia University Student Research Poster Presentations 2021. 36. https://digitalcommons.misericordia.edu/research_posters2021/36

Lee, D., & Yoon, S. N. (2021). Application of artificial intelligence-based technologies in the healthcare industry: Opportunities and challenges. *International Journal of Environmental Research and Public Health, 18*(1), 271. https://doi.org/10.3390/ijerph18010271

Luzzi, P. (2021). *Planetree patient care model.* Misericordia University Student Research Poster Presentations 2021. 49. https://digitalcommons.misericordia.edu/research_posters2021/49

McCarthy, C. P. (2016). Validation of the Empatica E4 wristband. In *IEEE EMBS international student conference (ISC)* (pp. 1–4). IEEE.

Minvielle, E. F. (2021). Current developments in delivering customized care: A scoping review. *BMC Health Services Research, 21,* 1–29.

Minvielle, E. W. (2014). Managing customization in health care: A framework derived from the services sector literature. *Health Policy, 117*(2), 216–227.

Mishra, V. K., Hoyt, R. E., Wolver, S. E., Yoshihashi, A., & Banas, C. (2019). Qualitative and quantitative analysis of patients' perceptions of the patient portal experience with OpenNotes. *Applied Clinical Informatics, 10*(1), 10–18.

Mostaghel, R. (2016). Innovation and technology for the elderly: Systematic literature review. *Journal of Business Research, 69*(11), 4896–4900.

Proclinical. (2022, June 9). *Who are the top 10 medical device companies in the world in 2022?* Retrieved July 17, 2023, from www.proclinical.com/blogs/2022-9/the-top-10-medical-device-companies-in-the-world-in-2022

Rodriguez, M. M., Casper, G., & Brennan, P. F. (2007). Patient-centered design: The potential of user-centered design in personal health records. *Journal of AHIMA, 78*(4), 44–46.

Sanchez Antelo, V., Szwarc, L., Paolino, M., Saimovici, D., Massaccesi, S., Viswanath, K., & Arrossi, S. (2022). A counseling mobile app to reduce the psychosocial impact of human papillomavirus testing: Formative research using a user-centered design approach in a low-middle-income setting in Argentina. *JMIR Formative Research, 6*(1), e32610.

Savage, L. G.-M. (2018). Digital health data and information sharing: A new frontier for health care competition. *Antitrust LJ, 82,* 593–621.

Stanford Byers Center for Biodesign. (2024). *Programs.* https://biodesign.stanford.edu/programs.html

Stanford Medicine 25. (n. d.). Retrieved July 17, 2023, from https://stanfordmedicine25.stanford.edu/the25.html

Tzenios, N. (2019). The determinants of access to healthcare: A review of individual, structural, and systemic factors. *Journal of Humanities and Applied Science Research, 2*(1), 1–14.

U.S. Food and Drug Administration. (2009, December). *Guidance for industry patient-reported outcome measures: Use in medical product development to support labeling claims.* U.S. Food and Drug Administration. www.fda.gov/media/77832/download

Walker, J., Leveille, S., Bell, S., Chimowitz, H., Dong, Z., Elmore, J. G., Delbanco, T., Fernandez, L., Fossa, A., Gerard, M., Fitzgerald, P., & Harcourt, K. (2019). OpenNotes after 7 years: Patient experiences with ongoing access to their clinicians' outpatient visit notes. *Journal of Medical Internet Research, 21*(5), e13876.

WHO. (2023, June 6). *Health innovation for impact*. Retrieved July 17, 2023, from www.who.int/teams/digital-health-and-innovation/health-innovation-for-impact#:~:text=WHO%20defines%20health%20innovation%20as,to%20accelerate%20positive%20health%20impact

Zou, J., & Schiebinger, L. (2021). Ensuring that biomedical AI benefits diverse populations. *EBioMedicine, 67.*

CHAPTER 14 ALERT: CONSIDERATIONS FOR INCORPORATION OF NEW INNOVATIONS IN HEALTHCARE

CHRISTY LENAHAN

The landscape of healthcare is in a state of constant change that is driven by consumer demand and technological innovation. Today's healthcare consumers are looking for high-quality, results-driven, personalized, convenient, and affordable healthcare (Bengston & McCanna, 2023); thus, new innovations in healthcare have focused on many of these demands. Some of these innovations, like remote patient monitoring, can be traced back to the 1960s but have been significantly improved through augmentation with artificial intelligence (AI) and machine learning. Other innovations, such as clustered regularly interspaced short palindromic repeats (CRISPR) technology and bioprinting for tissue engineering are newer to healthcare but demonstrate a promising future in addressing healthcare consumer demands.

Remote patient monitoring, which allows a clinician to monitor different aspects of a patient's health from remote locations such as their home, was initially used in 1961 when the National Aeronautics and Space Administration (NASA) utilized biosensors to measure the body temperature, respiratory rate and depth, and heart rate and rhythm of Astronaut Alan Shepard in the first U.S. manned suborbital space flight (NASA, 1961). Since 1961, remote patient monitoring has become more accessible, with several companies providing direct-to-consumer wearable health technology. These wearable health technologies include wristbands or watches that can monitor heart rate and rhythm, oxygen saturation, sleep patterns, handwashing effectiveness, and fall potential, as well as clothing that can measure muscle activity and motion tracking during physical exertion.

While these direct-to-consumer wearable health devices can be, and have been, used in healthcare, more sophisticated devices are dedicated to remote patient monitoring of persons with acute and chronic diseases in a variety of healthcare and nonhealthcare settings. Many of these devices incorporate AI and/or machine learning. AI, when integrated into remote patient monitoring devices, can evaluate symptoms and biomarkers in real time and assist clinicians in slowing and potentially stopping illness progression. Additionally, machine learning (a subset of AI) can improve patient care through rapid interpretation of complex datasets combined with the patient's unique characteristics, predicting a patient's potential for deterioration and enhancing healthcare decision-making through use of preprogrammed and learned evidence-based algorithms (Shaik et al., 2023).

An example of AI integration in remote patient monitoring is an AI-powered virtual health assistant that is able to converse with the patient being monitored, provide resources or advice as needed, and send positive reinforcement for consistent use of the remote patient monitoring system or encouragement when the patient is not compliant. One review demonstrated that over the course of 180 days, use of AI-enabled remote patient monitoring decreased blood pressure by 4.7 mmHg in patients with hypertension, decreased average blood glucose levels by 7.5 mg/dL in patients with diabetes, and over a period of 90 days decreased weight by 8.2 pounds in patients whose starting weight was greater than 286 pounds (Pundi et al., 2022).

While AI-augmented remote patient monitoring has shown significant benefits in improving patient health outcomes, there is a probability that in genetic diseases, technology such as CRISPR may be able to eliminate the disease process altogether. This technology allows researchers to manipulate the DNA of cells and has shown promising results in humans suffering from genetic diseases such as β-thalassemia and sickle cell disease, recessive dystrophic epidermolysis bullosa, and Duchenne muscular dystrophy (Abdelnour et al., 2021). In patients with β-thalassemia and sickle cell disease, CRISPR technology resulted in significant gene editing of bone marrow and blood cells and elimination of vasoocclusive episodes (Frangoul et al., 2021). In patients with recessive dystrophic epidermolysis bullosa, CRISPR technology resulted in a large proportion of corrected cells producing functional collagen (Bonafont et al., 2019). In one patient with Duchenne muscular dystrophy, the use of CRISPR technology resulted in successful correction of exon 44 deletions, a deletion seen in approximately 12% of patients with this type of muscular dystrophy (Min et al., 2019). Other disease processes in which CRISPR technology has shown some promise in animal studies include atherosclerosis, phenylketonuria, facioscapulohumeral muscular dystrophy, cystic fibrosis, ornithine transcarbamylase deficiency, primary hyperoxaluria type I, and hearing loss (Abdelnour et al., 2021); however, until the cost of therapy, which can run anywhere from 0.5 million to 2.125 million U.S. dollars, is decreased, expansive use of CRISPR technology is extremely limited (Gostimskaya, 2022).

Another promising innovation in healthcare includes the use of bioprinting for tissue engineering, which involves creating three-dimensional models of tissues or organs for repair or replacement using different types of bioink (Xie et al., 2020). The first and only successful implantation of bioprinted tissue in a human occurred in 2022 when a team from 3DBio Therapeutics performed an ear tissue implant in a 20-year-old woman using the patient's own cells (Corkill, 2022). Around the same time the ear implant occurred, researchers in Poland reported that they successfully implanted a bioprinted pancreas into a pig and were able to establish stable blood flow over a two-week period (Wszola et al., 2022). Laboratories all over the world are creating bioprinted tissues and organs, including multilayered skin, bones, muscle structures, blood vessels, retinal tissues, lung tissue capable of oxygen exchange, and even a "rabbit-sized" heart. Though none of these bioprinted tissues are approved for human use, it is estimated that the ability to transplant a full-sized three-dimensional bioprinted organ is only 20 to 30 years away, with smaller structures such as skin patches to assist in wound healing being just a few years away (Barber, 2023).

New innovations will continue to transform healthcare delivery and disease management. Extensive research has already provided evidence of the positive impact of AI-augmented remote patient monitoring on enhancing diagnostic accuracy and improving health outcomes. Simultaneously, the potential of CRISPR technology to mitigate the effects of specific genetic diseases has been widely recognized. Further, the need for human organ donation may be nonexistent in a few decades once bioprinting of tissue is perfected. Healthcare providers and consumers should embrace innovations that are patient-centered and focused on improving the human condition while imploring researchers and political leaders to ensure responsible and equitable implementation of these technologies.

References

Abdelnour, S. A., Xie, L., Hassanin, A. A., Zuo, E., & Lu, Y. (2021). The potential of CRISPR/Cas9 gene editing as a treatment strategy for inherited diseases. *Frontiers in Cell and Developmental Biology, 9*, 1–17. https://doi.org/10.3389/fcell.2021.699597

Barber, C. (2023, February 15). 3D-printed organs may soon be a reality: Looking ahead, we'll no need donor hearts. *Fortune.* https://fortune.com/well/2023/02/15/3d-printed-organs-may-soon-be-a-reality/

Bengston, N., & McCanna, L. (2023). *What today's healthcare consumers expect.* Huron Consulting Group Inc. www.huronconsultinggroup.com/insights/what-healthcare-consumers-expect

Bonafont, J., Menca, A., Garcia, M., Torres, R., Rodriguez, S., Carretero, M., Chacon-Solano, E., Modamio-Hoybjor, S., Marinas, L., Leon, C., Escamez, M. J., Hausser,

I., Rio, M. D., Murillas, R., & Larcher, F. (2019). Clinically relevant correction of recessive dystrophic eipderolysis bullosa by dual sgRNA CRISPR/Cas-9-mediated gene editing. *Molecular Therapy*, 27(5), 986–998. https://doi.org/10.1016/j.ymthe.2019.03.007

Corkill, B. (2022, June 3). *Lab-grown ear made from patient's own cells and successfully implanted.* IFLScience. www.iflscience.com/labgrown-ear-made-from-patients-own-cells-and-successfully-implanted-63933

Frangoul, H., Altshuler, D., Cappellini, M. D., Chen, Y., Domm, J., Eustace, B. K., Foell, J., de la Fuente, J., Grupp, S., Handgretinger, R., Ho, T. W., Kattamis, A., Kernytsky, A., Lekstrom-Himes, J., Li, A. M., Locatelli, F., Mapara, M. Y., de Montalembert, M., Rondelli, D., Sharma, A., . . . Corbacioglu, S. et al. (2021). CRISPR-Cas9 gene editing for sickle cell disease and β-thalassemia. *New England Journal of Medicine*, 384(3), 252–260. https://doi.org/10.1056/NEJMoa2031054

Gostimskaya, I. (2022). CRISPR-Cas9: A history of its discovery and ethical considerations of its use in genome editing. *Biochemistry, Biokhimiia*, 87(8), 777–788. https://doi.org/10.1134/S0006297922080090

Min, Y., Bassel-Duby, R., & Olson, E. N. (2019). CRISPR correction of Duchenne muscular dystrophy. *Annual Review of Medicine*, 70, 239–255. https://doi.org/10.1146/annurev-med-081117-010451

National Aeronautics and Space Administration. (1961, June 6). *Proceedings of a conference on results of the first U.S. manned suborbital space flight* (Report No. N64-80458). https://tothemoon.ser.asu.edu/files/mercury/mercury_redstone_3_results.pdf

Pundi, K., Turakhia, M., & Wurm, M. (2022). *Patient outcomes using remote patient monitoring.* ConnectAmerica. www.connectamerica.com/wp-content/uploads/2022/04/Patient-Outcomes-Using-RPM-Connect-America-and-100Plus.pdf

Shaik, T., Tao, A., Higgins, N., Li, L., Gururajan, X. Z., & Acharya, U. R. (2023). Remote patient monitoring using artificial intelligence: Current state, applications, and challenges. *WIREs Data Mining and Knowledge Discovery*, 13(2), e1485. https://doi.org/10.1002/widm.1485

Wszola, M., Klak, M., Berman, A., Kolodziejska, M., Bryniarski, T., Tymicki, G., Dobrzanski, T., Szkopek, D., Roszkowicz-Ostrowska, K., Wolinski, J., Dobrzyn, A., & Kaminski, A. (2022, June 4). *Bionic pancreas – 3D bioprinting of a bionic organ with a vascular system – results of transplantation in large animals* [Conference Session]. 2022 American Transplant Congress, Boston, MA. https://atcmeetingabstracts.com/abstract/bionic-pancreas-3d-bioprinting-of-a-bionic-organ-with-a-vascular-system-results-of-transplantation-in-large-animals/

Xie, Z., Gao, M., Lobo, A. O., & Webster, T. J. (2020). 3D bioprinting in tissue engineering for medical applications: The classic and the hybrid. *Polymers*, 12(8), 1717. https://doi.org/10.3390/polym12081717

Definition of Terms

Artificial intelligence (AI)– Utilization of computers and/or other machines to mimic tasks such as problem-solving and decision-making, which are normally done by a human.

Bioprinting – Three-dimensional printing of tissue or cells using bioink, which may consist of natural or synthetic materials that are compatible with biological stressors it may be exposed to.

Clustered regularly interspaced short palindromic repeats (CRISPR) technology – A type of technology that can be used to edit genes through precision cutting of DNA that is followed by a natural repair process.

Machine learning – A type of artificial intelligence that allows computers and/or other machines to learn without explicit programming. Machine learning may include use of known input and output data to predict future outputs or machine based grouping of data to find underlying or hidden patterns.

Remote patient monitoring – A type of healthcare that allows the clinician to monitor different aspects of a patient's health from remote locations such as their home.

INDEX

Note: Page numbers in *italics* indicate figures. Page numbers in **bold** indicate tables in the text, and references following "n" refer to notes.